Pharmacology

MEDCHARTS™

Tables and Summaries for Review

IMPORTANT NOTICE

Pharmacology

MEDCHARTS™

Tables and Summaries for Review

Kevin P. Rosenbach, M.D.
University of South Florida
Tampa, Florida

ILOC, Inc.
Publishers
New York
Granville

I dedicate this book to my parents, for putting the goal of education for their children above everything else. To my brothers and sister, for sharing their time with me when I could not do the same. To my friends, who endured the hardships and shared the joy of our education. And to my wife, for sticking by my side through medical school and residency.

Pharmacology: *MedCharts* Tables and Summaries for Review

1 2 3 4 5 6 7 8 9 0 DOHDOH 9 8 7 6 5 4 3

ISBN 1-882531-00-0

This book was set in Utopia by ILOC, Inc..
The editors were John Thornborough and Deborah Harvey.
The production supervisor was Diana Porter.
R. R. Donnelley & Sons was printer and binder.

Library of Congress Cataloging-in-Publication Data

Rosenbach, Kevin P. (Kevin Philip), 1963-
  Pharmacology : MedCharts : tables and summaries for review / Kevin
P. Rosenbach.
        p.   cm.
  Includes bibliographical references and index.
  ISBN 1-882531-00-0 (pbk.)
  1. Drugs--Tables. 2. Pharmacology--Tables.   I. Title.
  [DNLM: 1. Drugs--classification--tables. 2. Pharmacology--tables.
QV 38 R813p]
RM301. 12.R68   1993
615'.7--dc20
DNLM/DLC
for Library of Congress   92-49118
                                                          CIP

CONTENTS

6 ANTIBIOTICS (continued)

7 OTHER TOPICS   134

Preface

Pharmacology: MEDCHARTS Tables and Summaries for Review was written to help medical students master the complicated field of pharmacology. Information about many of the common drugs essential to a medical student is grouped by drug action and type. The mechanism of action, effects, routes of metabolism and excretion, efficacy, contraindications, resistance (with antibiotics), side effects, and toxicity all are included. Additional charts on drug interactions, arrhythmias, and prescription writing are also included in this book. The format, placement of information into charts, facilitates the learning and comparison of related drugs.

This is actually the third version of this book, but the first to be published and widely distributed. I wrote the first version while trying to learn pharmacology myself. Being frustrated with the complexity of pharmacology and the lack of easy-to-use learning materials, I began to make my own charts and to distribute them to my classmates. The second version was written while I was studying for the National Boards, Part I. I found these charts to be a valuable resource for the type of studying required to succeed on the Boards. This last (third) effort was written during my clinical year of medical school. I added additional information and drugs to augment the already detailed charts. I find it very rewarding that students from successive classes tell me they would not have passed the Pharmacology class or the pharmacology section of the National Boards without these charts.

Pharmacology: MEDCHARTS Tables and Summaries for Review is not meant to replace a formal class in pharmacology or a good textbook. Information in the charts is referenced to major pharmacology texts. I encourage you to check the references in order to extend your knowledge of the drugs you are studying. This book is a learning aid that is easy to use and packed with information to help you learn, understand, and remember pharmacology.

Kevin P. Rosenbach
1993

1 AUTONOMIC

1

CATECHOLAMINES and other β agonists	EPINEPHRINE [1]	NOREPINEPHRINE [2]
ADMINISTRATION	Infusion, Inhalation	Infusion
RECEPTORS (Mechanism)	α, β_1, β_2 (adrenal medulla) α - ITP inc BP° inc conc – $\alpha > \beta$ β - cAMP dec BP° dec conc – $\beta > \alpha$ (direct effect)	Predominantly α $\alpha > \beta_1$ No β_2 (direct acting)

EFFECTS Cardiovascular	(+) inotropic
	(+) chronotropic (tachycardia)
	    both increase CO
	Arrhythmia (dose depend)
	esp. w/ halogenated hydrocarbons
	inc oxygen demand
	    (don't use if heart problem)
		Dec HR (bradycardia)
		(reflex due to inc BP inc
		Vagal output)
		
		(+) inotropic
		(-) chronotropic (reflex)

Vascular
 	
Blood Pressure
	α • vasoconstrict
	    • stim mucous membs • small doses
	β_2 – vasodilate skeletal muscle
	Dose dependent
	Inc systolic BP° (pressor drug)
	Vasoconstrict, inc CO
	Slight dec diastolic BP°
	Peripheral resistance
	Pulse pressure – big inc,
	Mean Art P° – slight inc,
	Small dose – dec PR β,
	Large dose – inc PR
		Intense vasoconstrictor
		Inc systolic BP°
		Inc diastolic BP°
		Inc mean Art P° use to
		Used for shock because
		    inc BP°
		
		Inc peripheral resistance

Pulmonary	β_2 – bronchodilate (smooth muscle)
	    for acute asthma
	Acidosis, poor EPI response
	Large dose – apnea
	Give subcutaneously or inhale,
	    NOT IV
		Never use
		
		No β_2 action

Skeletal muscle	Inc contractility
	Inc release ACh
	Direct effect on myosin
	    • alleviate fatigue • inc muscle power
	    Myasthenia gravis	

Urinary System	Dec GFR (transient) Constrict BV – inc renin	Vasoconstricts kidney vessels
METABOLISM	Hyperglycemia Asthma Tx • inc blood sugar α • dec insulin β_2 • inc glucagon • inc glycogenolysis β_1 • inc lipolysis	Minor effect

USES	Acute asthma, anaphylaxis
	Topically – dec bleeding
	    (eosinopenia) (mucosa)
	Local anesthesia – inc duration (α)
	Mydriatic – dilation
	    Dec intraocular pressure
		Tx: Hypotensive state
		    can't be used for
		    prolonged time
		• Dec kidney function
		    (see Dopamine)

CONTRAINDICATIONS	Halothane, Cocaine, Hyperthyroidism, or Guanethione	

DOPAMINE [3]	ISOPROTERENOL [4]	TERTBUTALINE [5] ALBUTEROL	RITODRINE [6] (Yutopar®)
Infusion	Infusion, inhalation	Oral, Inhalation	IV
β_1 activity High dose α effects (direct)	Synthetic β_1 & β_2 activity (direct)	β_2 agonist Inc cAMP	β_2 agonist

(+) inotropic
(+) chronotropic
increase CO
 	
Lipolysis
	(+) inotropic
	(+) chronotropic as potent as EPI
	Inc HR, inc myocardial O_2 demand
	Can produce arrhythmia
		Asthma:
		  Oral – chronic
		  Inhale – acute
		
		Heart – minimal
		  effect
			Give IV until contractions stop, then give orally

inc systolic BP°
diastolic same
inc MAP
 	
Dec peripheral resistance at low dose
NO α
NO vasoconstriction
	β_2
	Greatest dec in peripheral resistance of all catecholamines
	
	Dec BP°
	
	Inc systolic BP°
	Dec diastolic BP°
	Dec MAP
		Dec BP° 10 mmHg
		
		Albuterol
		  Long duration 6 – 8 hr
		  Onset 30 – 45 min
			Dec BP°
			10 mmHg

	Asthma (inhalation) longer duration than EPI ISO = 1 hr EPI = 30 min	Asthma – bronchodilator can be inhaled with longer duration than ISO or EPI AL 4 - 6 hrs	Asthma (can be used, but is not)
		Tocolytic effect reduces uterine contractions prolongs gestation (all β_2 agonists)	Tocolytic effect most often used No effect on fetus
Dilates vessels to the kidney			
Enhances Na^+ excretion			Inc gestation by one month Can be used for asthma
Tx: Shock – OK prolonged use inc BP° by cardiac effect No vasoconstriction (no α) cardiogenic or septic shock	Asthma	Side effects • tremors in extremities • inc blood sugar • fasciculation (all β_2 agonists)	
	Digitalis MI – inc infarcted area		

BETA ADRENERGIC ANTAGONISTS	PROPRANOLOL [27]	TIMOLOL [28]	PINDOLOL [29]
ADMINISTRATION	Infusion, Oral	Eyedrops	
MODE OF ACTION	β_1 & β_2 (nonselective) blocker (competitive inhibitor) • dec HR (and CO) • dec BP° (lag) in hypertensives • NO effect with normotensives	β_1 & β_2 blocker Topical – eyedrops Long acting	β_1 & β_2 antagonist Partial α agonist
USE		Glaucoma: • dec intraocular P° • dec secretion of aqueous humor • No effect on outflow of fluid Does not change ability to focus (like Pilocarpine)	Intrinsic sympatho-mimetic activity Doesn't lower heart rate No reduction of exercise ability of normal people Does not dec CO

USE (Propranolol column):

Quinidine-like activity, inc refractory period of SA and AV node (dec conduction velocity)
Dec automaticity of AV node
Peripheral resistance may not dec
Dec CO and dec HR causing a dec BP° (block vasoconstriction)
• Angina pectoris (depressed ST seg) poor oxygenation
• inc exercise tolerance
Heart improves by dec oxygen demand
• dec cardiac rate (-) inotropic
• dec cardiac force (-) chronotropic
• longer systole time
May effect blood redistribution
ST depression disappears
MI – catechol leak out, more damage
IV injection of β blockers: • dec damage
• dec risk of 2nd MI
Asthma – don't give, use Aminophylline in emergencies
Glycogenolysis and glucagon release blocked
Diabetic: dec blood sugar – hypoglycemia
Tx: prophylaxis chronic migraine
Tx: Thyrotoxicosis – inc synthesis of adren receptors
– inc symp activity
Thyroid Storm IV β blocker
Does NOT treat – dec symp effects
Block lipolysis but: • inc triglycerides • inc LDLs • dec HDL
Glaucoma: • dec intraocular P°
• dec secretion of aqueous humor
Do NOT abruptly withdraw β blockers – arrythmia

Catech	Control	β blocker
ISO		(β)
EPI		(α, β)
NE		(α)

Contraindicated with:
1. Diabetics (hypoglycemic)
2. Asthmatics (bronchodilation blocked)
3. CHF (dec, impaired contractility)
4. Raynaud's (vasoconstrict, dec flow)

Pindolol column (TX):
TX
• Angina
• Hypertension
• Glaucoma
• Athletes with hypertension

Only beta blocker that is NOT a cardiac depressant

NADOLOL[30]	METOPROLOL[31] ATENOLOL ACEBUTOLOL	ESMOLOL[32]	LABETALOL[33]
	Oral	IV	Oral
Nonselective β blocker (β_1 & β_2) Long acting	All three β_1 selective (cardioselective)	β_1 selective Short acting	α, β_1 & β_2 blocker (sympatholytic) β > α 3:1 Long duration
	Can be used in: 1. Asthmatics (carefully) (NO β_2 block) (NO effect on bronchodilation) 2. Diabetics with hypertension (NO block on glyco-genolysis or glucagon release) Dec BP° • Antiarrhythmic Very high doses • spillover (blocks β_2 also) ATENOLOL • does NOT inhibit renin release (most others do)	Anesthesia	Antihypertensive Tx: Hypertension • dec BP° by dec HR Can develop postural hypotension • blocks vasoconstriction Side effects: (anti-α) 1. Postural hypotension 2. Blocks normal sexual activity

HYPOTENSIVE ACTION (dec BP°)
β BLOCKERS • dec CO, dec HR
  • most dec renin release
  • NO effect on peripheral resistance
  • NO orthostatic hypotension
α BLOCKERS • dec peripheral resistance
  Orthostatic hypotension occurs
ANTIARRHYTHMIC ACTION – β BLOCKERS
Dec Arrhythmias that are:
  1. Paroxysmal Supraventricular Tachycardia (PAT (atrial))
  2. Exercise arrhythmias
Dec Wolff-Parkinson-White
Poor effect on ventricular arrhythmias
  • unless caused by large inc catecholamines
    (pheochromocytoma and neuroblastoma)

ADRENERGIC alpha agonists (direct)	PHENYLEPHRINE [7] (Neosynephrine®)	OXYMETAZOLINE [8] (Neosynephrine-12®) (Afrin®) nose drops	METHOXAMINE [9]	NOREPINEPHRINE [10]	PROPADRINE [11]
ADMINISTRATION	Nasal spray	Nasal spray	Infusion		
MODE OF ACTION	α_1 agonist Parenteral use Topical (nose drops) (direct)	α_1 agonist Topical only (direct)	α agonist (direct)	α_1 agonist	α agonist (mixed acting)
USE	Nasal decongestant Lasts 3 – 4 hrs Causes an intense vasoconstriction with NO inc HR Tx: Incontinence	Nose drops • lasts 10 hrs	Nose drops • inc BP°	See Catecholamines	
EFFECTS	Parenterally • inc peripheral resistance • inc BP° • dec HR (reflex bradycardia) NOT inactivated by COMT Vasodilation if used too frequently	Vasoconstriction if used too often, receptors desensitize, dec effectiveness Vasodilation if used too frequently	Parenterally • inc peripheral resistance • inc HR • inc BP° (vasoconstrict α action)		Vasoconstriction

ADRENERGIC alpha and beta agonists (direct & mixed)	EPHEDRINE [12]	DOBUTAMINE [13]	METARAMINOL [14]	CLONIDINE [15]
ADMINISTRATION	Oral	IV	Injection	
MODE OF ACTION	α, β_1, β_2 (like EPI, less potent) Promotes NE release Tachyphylaxis (quick tolerance) Long acting pressor Vasoconstrictor (mixed acting) Tachycardia – stimulate heart	Selective β_1 agonist (direct)	α - Vasopressor β_1 - Heart stimulant (mixed)	α_2 agonist Feedback inhibition of norepinephrine Inhibits release of norepinephrine
EFFECTS	Inc systolic BP° Inc diastolic BP° Inc Heart Rate CNS: Good penetration Mild stimulant, like amphetamine • inc alertness • insomnia • dec fatigue Inc skeletal muscle activity Used for Myasthenia Gravis along with anticholinesterase Prophylaxis of chronic asthma – β_2 (bronchodilate) Urology – (α) control incontinence, internal sphincter, 3 – 4 hr	Short duration • can be used for • acute MI • heart surgery Inc cardiac contractility ((+) inotropic) Inc heart rate ((+) chronotropic) Inc cardiac output No change in peripheral resistance Acute basis only	Tx: Shock (if can't give dopamine infusion) – one shot Tx: Incontinence	

Meuller's muscle in eyelid
α agonist – opens eyelid
α blocker – closes eyelid

ALPHA ADRENERGIC ANTAGONIST	PHENOXYBENZAMINE [21]	PHENTOLAMINE [22]
ADMINISTRATION	Oral	Parenterally
MODE OF ACTION	α_1 & α_2 blocker Transient dec BP° No heart effect (β_1) Prodrug cyclizes to active cyclic amine Covalent bond (irreversible)	α_1 & α_2 block Transient dec BP° No heart effect Short duration (4 hrs) Reversible (competitive inhibitor)
USES	Long duration: 1 – 2 days Onset time: 2 hr Related to nitrogen mustard Tx: hypertension (Pheo) • blocks vasoconstriction • dec peripheral resistance	Old test for Pheochromocytoma • inject in supine position • if dec 35 mm systolic • if dec 25 mm diastolic •indicates Pheo
EFFECTS (all alpha blockers cause EPI reversal)	Causes EPI reversal Catechl Control α block ISO β EPI β NE dec Tx: of impotence Urologist; Tx: • Paraplegics, to treat reflex inc BP° due to urination • Neurogenic vascular dysfunction • Premature closure of internal sphincter • Benign prostatic hypertrophy	Vasodilator: (inc NE release) Impotent men • inject into penis • erection 1 hr Frostbite Peripheral vascular disease NOT effective for heart treatment
SIDE EFFECTS	Postural hypotension (blocks postural sympathetic reflex) Male sexual dysfunction • block ejaculation • retrograde ejaculation EPI reversal • α blocked • β allowed to predominate NE dec effect (α) Reflex tachycardia (dec PR, dec BP°) **TOLERANCE** block α_2 – inc NE build up NE – overcome α_1 block	Postural hypotension Male sexual dysfunction EPI reversal Reflex tachycardia Tolerance

PRAZOSIN [23] (Minipress®) TERAZOSIN TRIMAZOSIN	ERGOT ALKALOIDS[24] Ergotamine Dihydroergotamine Ergonovine	CLONIDINE [25]	YOHIMBINE [26]
Oral			
α_1 blocker (selective)	α blocker Fungus of rye grain Independently constricts smooth muscle, therefore can still inc PR	α_2 "agonist" Similar effect as an α_1 blocker, Feedback inhibition of NE (see antihypertens)	α_2 blocker (dec feedback) Enhance sympathetic activity by inc NE release
Effective in Tx of hypertension Used only if first drug failed	Migraine headaches – given in prodrome Constricts smooth muscle of blood vessels acute attack Stops vasospasm		
First dose effect (reduce first dose to ¼ and give at bedtime) • blood pooling • bradycardia Vasodilation • dec BP°	Ergonovine – inc smooth musc contraction in the uterus (Oxytocic) St Anthony's Fire Vasoconstricts Uterine contraction Hallucinations		
Less postural hypotension Relatively NO adverse effect on male sexuality EPI reversal NO reflex tachycardia (not acting at α_2), making PRAZOSIN the D.O.C.	Vasospasm – constricts Can cause 1. Coronary occlusion 2. If give too much, dec blood supply to digits, • Gangrene • Raynaud's disease patients, must be careful Direct effect on smooth muscle, despite its α receptor block • smooth musc contracts • inc BP°		

ADRENERGIC REUPTAKE INHIBITORS and DEPLETORS	COCAINE [34]	IMIPRAMINE [35]
ADMINISTRATION	Inhaled, Smoked, IV	
MODE OF ACTION	Blocks reuptake of catecholamines via Na^+/K^+ ATPase pump Inc NE at receptor site	Blocks reuptake Tricyclic antidepressants
USE	ENT surgery Drug abuse Topical or Parenteral • dec bleeding (VC) Inc adrenergic response Best local anesthetic because it also causes vasoconstriction Stimulates entire cerebral spinal axis	Psych use: antidepressant
SIDE EFFECTS	Can cause arrhythmia and ventricular fibrillation Inc BP°, cause stroke • inc diastolic P° • inc systolic P° CNS – enters rapidly • euphoria • seizures • inc Body T° (pyogenic) Potentiates the effects of NE and EPI Can cause tissue necrosis due to vasoconstriction Cocca leaves – reduce appetite IV (high dose): • Respiration depression (stop breathing) Freebase – Crack NO antidote	

BRETYLIUM [36]	RESERPINE [37]	GUANETHIDINE [38] (8 membered ring)
	Oral	IV
Blocks release of Catechols	Depletor NE depletion by blocking Mg^{++} ATPase Vesicle reuptake of cytoplasmic NE (chemical sympathectomy)	

Antiarrhythmic	For Hypertension
	• dec BP°
	• dec cardiac output
	• dec peripheral resistance
	
	Long acting, 1 dose/day because depletes NE
	
	RES + Indirect acting adrenergic agonist
	gives a dec response
	
	RES + Direct acting adrenergic agonist
	gives a normal response of the direct agonist
		Use for hypertension only if other drugs fail
		• dec BP°
		• dec cardiac rate
		
		Must be taken up by Na$^+$/K$^+$ ATPase (therefore, drug can be blocked by Cocaine)
		
		When first given IV
		• transient inc NE
		    inc BP°
		• then dec NE
		    dec BP°

	Nightmares
	Bradycardia
	Peptic ulcers
	• inc parasympathetic stim
	• inc GI activity, secretion
	Suicidal depression
	
	NE synthesis continues but it can't be stored in vesicles, becomes depleted
	
	Dec sympathetic, accentuates parasympathetic
	
	Orthostatic hypotension not a major problem because CNS depressed, also
		Bradycardia
		
		Severe hypotension
		    Orthostatic hypotension
		
		Blocks ejaculation
		
		Chronic use:
		• Supersensitivity
		• α and β receptors become Hypersensitive
		    • inc number receptors
		    • inc sensitivity
		
		Contraindicated with:
		1. EPI
		2. MAO inhibitors

ADRENERGIC agonists indirect acting	RESERPINE [16]	AMPHETAMINE [17]	METHYL [18] AMPHETAMINE	HYDROXY [19] AMPHETAMINE	TYRAMINE [20]
ADMINISTRATION		Oral	Oral, "ice" , "speed"		(Prototype)
MODE OF ACTION	Indirect, Depletion • prevents NE from reentering vesicle • block Mg^{++}/ATPase	Indirect α agonist, some $β_1$ Releases NE, dopamine, or 5-HT from nerves	Indirect Releases NE	Indirect	Indirect Promotes NE release
USE	Tx: Hypertension • to dec BP° Long acting • dec CO, dec PR		Drug abuse	Ophthalmic • Mydriatic	
EFFECTS	Chemical sympathectomy Deplete NE from neurons (CNS and PNS) If give with an indirect acting drug – get decreased response If give with a direct acting drug – get No effect Dec BP° • get tachycardia • then bradycardia after depletion CNS • sedation • depression • Parkinsonism Inc GI motility May cause nightmares NE can be synthesized, but can't be stored or released	Vasculature & heart Small dose • prevent sleep 24 hr • max = 36 hr Stimulates entire cerebral spinal axis, inc alertness Skeletal Muscle • inc contractility • inc athletic performance • abolish fatigue Raise BP° , Inc HR Attention Deficit Syndrome (4 - 15 years old), Now use (Ritalin®) Methylphenidate Depress appetite (for 2 weeks then returns) tolerance Abuse – causes strokes, give α and β blockers – arrhythmogenic Increased excretion in acidic urine	Very lipid soluble gets into CNS easily Compare w/ AMPH • high solubility • long duration	Polar • not soluble • little CNS activity	Tachyphylaxis Contraindicated: 1. MAO Inhibitors (Parkinson's disease therapy) Inc pressor effect (inc NE) because of dec break-down of NE 2. Cocaine blocks its uptake resulting in NO change because no NE is released 3. Reserpine (same as cocaine)

Psychic and Physical Dependence

Contraindicated with Cardiovascular disease or MAO inhibitors

CHOLINERGIC and PARASYMPATHETIC AGONISTS and BLOCKERS	ATROPINE[39] (ACh blocker)	NICOTINE[40] (blocker) CURARE	CARBACHOL[41] (ACh Agonist)	METHACHOLINE[42] (Agonist)	BETHANECHOL[43] (Agonist)	PILOCARPINE[44] (Agonist)
MODE OF ACTION	Muscarinic receptor blocker	Nicotinic receptor blocker NIC: Initially stimulates receptor CUR: blocker	Insensitive to AChE • longer lasting Mimics ACh at muscarinic receptor and nicotinic receptor	Slight resistance to AChE Pure muscarinic agonist NO effect on ganglia or skeletal muscle	Muscarinic agonist Total AChE resistant	Only one used as muscarinic agonist Naturally occurring alkaloid
USE	See CHOLINERGIC ANTAGONISTS	See CHOLINERGIC ANTAGONISTS	1° use: Eyedrops • constrict pupil Glaucoma • stop eye bleeding	NOT used clinically	Stimulate: Bladder (atonia) GI tract Esophageal reflux	Does all things that are due to inc parasympathetic Causes miosis Dec BP°
	Parasymp Symp Presyn ACh ACh Postsyn ACh NE Atropine (Muscarinic) Curare Nicotine (Nicotinic)		Side Effects (IV) • taken up by tissue • need large dose for effect • this dose tends to be toxic More potent as a Ganglionic stimulant (Nicotinic)	Longer lasting	No (-) inotropic No (-)chronotropic	For Tx: Glaucoma • dec intraocular P° • Narrow angle, pupil constricts • Wide angle, pores in Canal of Schlemm mesh become rounder Do NOT use systemic enters the CNS Change focusing ability Atropine Poisoning Test (-) NO effect = atropine poisoning (+) Miosis = neurologic problem

ACETYLCHOLINE

Affects Parasympathetic NS: • dec HR • Miosis • Accommodation changes • Short lived
Cardiovascular System
Muscarinic receptors in blood vessels that are not innervated by Symp and Parasymp NS
Extremely sensitive – marked dec in BP° without effect on HR
Low dose ACh – dec BP°, no change in HR (due to vasodilation)
High dose ACh – dec BP° and dec HR (and dec contraction)

ACETYL-CHOLINESTERASE INHIBITORS (REVERSIBLE)	PHYSOSTIGMINE [45]	NEOSTIGMINE [46]	CARBARYL [47] (SEVIN°)	EDROPHONIUM [48]	THA [49] (Tetrahydroamino-acridine)
ADMINISTRATION	Oral, Subcutaneous, IM	Parenterally		Parenterally	
MODE OF ACTION	(reversible AChE inhibitor)	(reversible)	(reversible)	(reversible)	Long duration AChE inhibitor
Potentiate ACh All AChE inhibitors increase parasympathetic effects by inc ACH in the synaptic cleft	Not charged – gets into CNS Competitive inhibitor with ACh for AChE receptors Ties up enzyme Inc effect of ACh since ACh is present longer	Resembles ACh in structure – ties up the enzyme Does NOT go into CNS (charged) Competitive inhibitor of AChE receptor Direct action on nicotinic receptor	Competitive inhibitor of AChE	Competitive inhibitor Block anionic site Simple interference	
USE	Miotic agent in glaucoma use with Pilocarpine Atropine poisoning antidote • inc ACh competes with Atropine Alzheimer's (short acting)	Atonic GI or bladder (MUSC) Myasthenia Gravis (NIC) NEO itself will not affect BP° or HR NEO + ACh: • dec BP° • dec HR	Pesticides	Dx: Myasthenia Gravis Antagonist to curare-like agents	Alzheimer's disease

AChE INHIBITORS (Irreversible)	DFP [50] (Isoflurophate)	ECHOTHIOPHATE [51]	PARATHION (P=S) PARAOXON (P=O) [52]	MALATHION [53]	SOMAN (GD) SARIN (GB) [54]	R_1, O, P, R_2, X ORGANO PHOSPHATE [55]
LIPID SOLUBLE	Very lipid soluble	NOT lipid soluble	Very lipid soluble	Very lipid soluble	Very lipid soluble	Some are prodrugs with P=S bond that is converted to P=O by metabolism and becomes active
	Combines with esteratic site only (phosphate group)	Only charged organophosphate not well absorbed • water soluble	More soluble because P=S Metabolized to P=O (activation)	P=S more soluble	SOMAN $T_{1/2}$ = 1O sec Very toxic	
USE	Glaucoma • oil drops Effect is miosis	Glaucoma • water soluble	Insecticides	Insecticides	Nerve gas	• Irreversible • Lipid soluble • Volatile • Absorbed through skin Long term neurological effects: • Paresthesia • Periph deficit • Dying back
EFFECTS	Effects of all depend upon route of entry. Different sequence, same symptoms: Nausea and vomiting Cramps (GI motility) Diarrhea Inc salivation Sweating	**EYES** Accommodation spasms Blurred vision Miosis	**SKIN** Muscle fasciculation **INHALED** Bronchial constriction Inc mucus secretion	**CNS** Confusion Delirium Hallucination Dec body T° Dec BP° Stimulation followed by paralysis	**DEATH** • Resp failure • Cardiovasc failure	

TREATMENT OF ORGANOPHOSPHATE POISONING

1. Atropine (muscarinic blocker)
   • counters all autonomic effects (muscarinic)   • antagonizes most CNS effects (muscarinic)
   • does NOT affect skeletal muscle (nicotinic) – paralysis   • can't block nicotinic receptors (still have skeletal muscle fasciculations and resp. distress)

2. Oximes (Pralidoxime)   • reacts with inhibited enzyme to pull inhibitor off
   (2 – PAM)   • restores enzyme activity (if before aging)   • can't be used prophylactically
   Aging (loss of one R group to form a monoalkyloid)   • oxine reaction NO longer possible   (irreversible)
   • most age in 6 – 24 hours (some (SOMAN) age in 10 seconds)

3. Carbamate cholinesterase inhibitors – not reversed by oxines (Pralidoxime)
   • oxines may make the situation worse

CHOLINERGIC ANTAGONISTS (blockers)	ATROPINE [56]	SCOPOLAMINE [57]	PIRENZEPINE [58]
MODE OF ACTION	Competitive antagonist to ACh Nonselective muscarinic antagonist Doesn't uniformly inhibit Sequence: 1st – Salivary gland (sensitive) dry mouth 2nd – Dryness of respiratory secretions and sweating 3rd – Loss of accommodation (cycloplegia) 4th – GI and bladder	Like Atropine except sedation at lower doses • Bradycardia • NO delirium More potent Shorter duration (MUSC antagonist)	Selective M_1 antagonist M_1 is GI selective
USE	Pupils dilate, Heart effects at higher dose, Paralysis of GI tract and bladder Tx: Parkinson's disease, Traveler's diarrhea, motion sickness **OPHTHALMIC** • Cycloplegia (loss of accommodation) • Mydriasis, contraindicated with glaucoma **CNS** • Inc dose – agitated, restless, delirium • inc Body T°, dec sweating • Elderly very sensitive, esp those who exercise • Antitremor (central) • Antidepressants have an atropine-like effect **HEART** • Initially dec HR, then inc HR • CNS – Cardiac inhib center very sensitive to Atropine First inc vagal tone: dec HR With time or higher dose, blocks vagus at receptor sites: inc HR Lower dose – inc Vagal tone: dec HR **BP:** • Oral, IM : NO effect • IV: inc peripheral resistance • Direct vasodilation on small vessels **GI TRACT:** antispasmodic **SECRETION** • dec Bronchodilation and salivary secretions • dec Gastric secretions • dec sweat gland secretion **PROPHYLAXIS** • Motion sickness • Preanesthesia to dry respiratory secretions • MI for sinus node bradycardia • Antidote to Atropine poisoning is Physostigmine • Test: Pilocarpine in eye, not constrict pupil, then ATR poisoning	**TREAT (SERUM)** • Motion sickness – transderm scopol • Amnestic, used during delivery – sedation – temporary amnesia **SIDE EFFECT** • Blurred vision • Cycloplegia • Dry mouth **HEART** • Only get dec HR (only CNS effect) • CANNOT give high enough dose to block receptors at heart • Only bradycardia (NO inc HR like Atropine)	Dec gastric acid Dec effect on gastric acid secretion (peptic ulcer) About as effective as H_2 inhibitor (Cimetidine + agonist)

GANGLIONIC BLOCKERS (cholinergic antagonists)	NICOTINE [59]	TRIMETHAPHAN [60]	HEXAMETHONIUM [61]	MECAMYLAMINE [62]
MODE OF ACTION	Stimulate receptors in ganglia and skeletal muscle CNS • Inc resp • nausea • vomiting Blocks transmission at sympathetic and parasympathetic ganglia NO clinical uses Initially: inc BP°, inc HR Inhibit ADH release	Ganglionic blocker (nicotinic) Short acting IV drip Hypertensive Emerg • can titrate to maintain a level	True ganglionic blocker (NIC) (autonomic ganglia only) NOT other nicotinic sites Blocks Ca^{++} channel 2 charged groups Doesn't get into CNS Competitive inhibition (reversible) NO initial stimulation	Ganglionic blocker (nicotinic) Used for hypertension Block both parasympathetic and sympathetic
EFFECTS	Hard to predict effect • Low dose – stimulate all the ganglia • High dose 2° depolarization causes desensitization, dec BP°, dec HR, vasodilation HEART RATE depends upon how it is administered SIDE EFFECTS Nausea, vomiting, paralysis, dec respiration, inc BP°		Selective ganglia blocking DOES NOT block skeletal muscle Block symp and parasymp effect depends on the time of the system blocks GI motility Inc HR dec BP° Mydriasis Dec sweating	(like Hexamethonium) Dec GI motility Inc HR Dec BP°
			All dominant control is 1° cholinergic (parasym) except the blood vessels (symp) Same effect as Atropine plus a dec in BP°, it blocks dominant control whether parasympathetic or sympathetic	

2 CARDIAC

GENERAL INFORMATION ABOUT CARDIAC GLYCOSIDES [68]

1. Direct Action: Restores cardiac function curve
   (+) Inotropy
   Inhibits Na^+/K^+ ATPase → Inc Na^+ → Inc Intracellular $[Ca^{++}]$ → Inc force of contraction
2. Indirect Action: (+) Inotropy, Inc CO, Relieves compensatory mechanisms which result in: Dec HR, Inc renal perfusion, Dec water retention

EGG
1. Vagomimetic: Dec HR (bradycardia), Dec conduction velocity through AV node (Inc conduction velocity in atria), used as antiarrhythmic – mediated by ACh (blocked by Atropine)
2. T Wave shape change – affects repolarization
3. PQ interval prolonged – Dec conduction AV node

VAGOMIMETIC ACTION
Dec HR, Inc PQ interval (M = muscarinic receptor)
   ACh + M ↔ AChM → Inc intracellular $[K^+]$ → More (–), hyperpolarizes → Inc time to threshold → Dec HR

NONAUTOMATIC CELLS
Faster ØO, Inc dv/dt → Inc conduction velocity, Inc K^+ perm (open channels) → hyperpolarizes cell, more Na^+ channels available,
Inc conduction velocity, Inc AP size, Dec time, shortening of refractory period, atrial fibers can drive faster, atrial tachycardia and fibrillation

TREATMENT
Glycosides are used to treat tissue with vagal input: Low dose – vagomimetic (parasymp), Dec HR, affect atrial and AV nodal function more be-cause of richer cholinergic innervation
1. PAT: Glycosides prophylaxis, sensitive to vagal stimulation
2. Supraventricular or atrial arrhythmias, flutters, or fibrillations: Glycosides Dec AV conduction, (Dec PQ), protects ventricles, ventricular ectopic foci may develop, arrhythmia. Tx: electric cardioversion
3. PVT (paradoxical ventricular tachycardia) Quinidine – an antiarrhythmic/local anesthetic, suppresses arrhythmia by dec # P waves, but more reach the AV node → paradoxical, Inc ventricular rate (Inc QRS), therefore, pretreat with digitalis: Prevents PVT by suppressing AV conduction (Dec QRS)

CARDIAC GLYCOSIDES	DIGOXIN [68]	DIGITOXIN [70]	OUABAIN [71]
ADMINISTRATION	Oral, more water soluble, absorbed best in capsules with (12' OH) hydroalcoholic vehicle	Oral, more lipid soluble, better (No OH)	Emergency treatment of cardiac failure only
Peak Levels Peak Effect Plasma Prt Bd	2 – 3 hrs 4 – 6 hrs 25%	3 – 6 hrs 6 – 12 hrs 90%	Rapid onset Short duration
Quinidine Interaction	Dec renal clearance	Inc T$_{1/2}$ Displace from protein, Pretreat before QUIN	
Metabolism / Excretion	Excreted unchanged into urine	Hepatic metabolism, excreted into gut, can be reabsorbed	
T$_{1/2}$	1.7 days May form inactive metabolite, dihydrodigoxin	7 days	

	Inhib Na$^+$/K$^+$ ATPase, Na$^+$/Ca^{++} exchange → Inc [Ca^{++}] → Inc force Shortened AP, Dec ventricular rate by inc ERP of conducting tissue Inc dv/dt = Inc force of contraction, Dec LVESV = better ejection, Dec LVEDV = Dec heart size & Dec preload, Dec Na$^+$ retention, Inc O$_2$ efficiency, better perfusion, Dec symp = Dec HR, Dec tone, Dec PR, Dec BP° = Dec afterload Glycosides may inc atrial rate, but dec ventricular HR by depressing the AV node, vagomimetic effect is blocked by atropine – brief period of prolonged AP with membrane rest potential followed by long period of shortened AP with dec membrane rest potential – sensitizes the carotid sinus (baroreceptors, Inc BP°) – sensitizes the AV node to ACh
SIDE EFFECTS	GI: nausea, vomiting, diarrhea, anorexia, CNS: Stim central chemoreceptors – vomiting, giddiness, color vision changes, convulsions, pain, delirium, hallucinations, skin rash, gynecomastia
TOXICITY	1. Cardiotoxicity: arrhythmia, tachycardia, fibrillation, bigeminy, Inc Na$^+$, Inc Ca^{++} → PVC. Tx toxicity with: LIDOCAINE and PHENYTOIN 2. Diuretic + glycosides → Inc toxicity. Dec K$^+$ → induce toxicity, because more glycoside binds to ATPase → depolarization and toxicity 3. Catecholamines: (+) chronotropic, (+) inotropic, potentiate toxicity → arrhythmia, activates slow Ca^{++} channels – phosphorylates them to open longer → Inc Ca^{++} induced toxicity. An Inc K$^+$ → Dec inhibition activity of glycosides (competitively inhibit digitalis), can be used to Tx digitalis toxicity
CONTRAINDICATED	Hyperkalemia or hypokalemia (diuretics), hypercalcemia, catecholamines (Isoproterenol), Wolff-Parkinson-White disease (AV shunt) is made worse

ALTERNATIVES TO GLYCOSIDES	AMRINONE [74] (Bipyridine)	DOBUTAMINE [75] PRENALTEROL	SALBUTAMOL [76] PIRBUTEROL	NITROGLYCERIN [77]
USE	Heart failure Wolff-Parkinson-White	β_1 agonist Heart failure, CHF emergency Tx	β_2 agonist Heart failure	Acute heart failure
ADMINISTRATION	Oral Short Term, $T_{1/2}$ = 2 – 3 hr	Parenterally – IV Intermittent		Skin or Sublingual Absorbed quickly, short duration
MECHANISM	Phosphodiesterase blocker → Inc cAMP → Inc [Ca⁺⁺] (+) Inotropic Inc dp/dt No membrane depolarization, safer	1. Inc cAMP → Inc [Ca⁺⁺] (+) Inotropic Less arrhythmogenic Less tendency to inc HR 2. Dec preload by venodilation (veins)	Dec afterload by vasodilation (arteries)	Vasodilate and venodilate 1. Venodilation causes dramatic dec of congestion, dec preload 2. Vasodilation causes dec afterload → Dec oxygen demand Redistributes flow to ischemic areas
SIDE EFFECTS	Nausea Vomiting → ion imbalance Muscle contractions	**PROBLEM WITH CHRONIC USE** 1. Tachyphylaxis, rapid tolerance Down regulate receptors (Must Wean Off Drug) 2. May inc HR → Inc O_2 demand → CHF Angina patients – may cause an angina attack Ischemic heart patients – may cause arrhythmia		**VENOUS POOLING CAUSES** • Hypotension • Dizziness • Weakness • Spastic angina • Headache, meningeal dilation • Flushing • Oxidize Hb → MHb MHb can be used to dec cyanide poisoning

---

NON-AUTOMATIC CELLS
1. Inc dv/dt: Inc AP size
   Dec duration AP
   Hyperpolarizes: Inc conduction velocity,
   Inc frequency, Dec refractory time,
   Dec HR – Drug; CARDIAC GLYCOSIDES
2. Dec dv/dt: Inc duration AP
   Inc refractory time (Prolong)
   Drugs: ANTIARRHYTHMICS,
   QUINIDINE (CARDIAC GLYCOSIDES in
   automatic cells)

METHYLXANTHINE ANALOGS
Similar to Bipyridine, less tachycardia,
less arrhythmia
Contraindicated: Angina

ANTI HYPERTENSIVES	VASODILATORS [63]	DIURETICS [64]
DRUGS	HYDRALAZINE MINOXIDIL SODIUM NITROPRUSSIDE DIAZOXIDE	HYDROCHLOROTHIAZIDE FUROSEMIDE SPIRONOLACTONE
	Inc HR and fluid volume Inc renal blood flow HYDRALAZINE Vasodilate (directly) Inc HR (reflex tachycardia), Dec BP° USE Preeclampsia (toxemia of pregnancy) (chronic) SIDE EFFECTS Ortho hypotension, reflex tachycardia, Na^+ and H_2O retention, headaches, palpitations UNIQUE SYMPTOMS Lupus-like syndrome, rheumatoid arthritis. Avoid if have MI MINOXIDIL Similar to hydralazine SIDE EFFECTS Hypertrichosis (inc hair growth) (chronic use), fluid retention, others above NO orthostatic hypotension Na NITROPRUSSIDE (hypertensive emergency) Short acting, IV drip, good vasodilator. Make up fresh and protect from light. Drug of choice DIAZOXIDE (hypertensive emergency) NOT a diuretic, powerful vasodilator. Looks like thiazide, but causes Na^+ retention	DUAL EFFECT 1. Initially: dec CO by inc Na^+ excretion 2. Then: dec blood vessel sensitivity (remain relaxed) With time, inc in blood volume REFLEX • Dec blood volume · Inc renin · Inc angiogenesis Give β blocker to stop sympathetic stimulation of renin (Propranolol) BETA BLOCKERS NO orthostatic hypotension PROBLEM K^+ loss (esp thiazides) ∴ supplement K^+

Calcium Channel Blockers

VERAPAMIL
- Dec BP°, Dec HR
- Affects both heart &
  blood vessels (relax)
- Use: cardiac arrhythmias

NIFEDIPINE
- Selective, acts on blood vessels
- Dec BP°, Inc HR (reflex)
- Sublingual route
- Sometimes hypertensive emergency

DILTIAZEM
- Cross between VER and NIF
- More cardiac effects

SYMPATHETIC BLOCKERS [65]	ACE INHIBITORS [66]	CNS (Effectors) INHIBITORS [67]
β Blockers – PROPRANOLOL α Block – PRAZOSIN (α_1) Nerve Term Block – RESERPINE – GUANETHIDINE Gang Block – TRIMETHAPHAN	CAPTOPRIL (has S) ENALAPRIL (prodrug) (has no S)	CLONIDINE α Methyl DOPA (Aldomet®)

β BLOCKERS
(by dec CO)
• Well tolerated
• NO sign of orthostatic hypotension
• NO sexual dysfunction
• Produces feeling of weakness
 	
PROBLEMS WITH
• Asthmatics
• Preexisting cardiac insufficiency
• Circulatory problems (Raynaud's)
• Diabetics
 	
WITHDRAWAL – rapid – arrhythmia
CO   Delayed BP° response.
BP°   Inc PR, gradually
PR   comes back down
 	
BLACKS
Hypertensive resistant, give diuretics
 	
α BLOCKERS (by dec PR)
• NO reflex tachycardia
• Orthostatic hypotension
(e.g. Prazosin)
 	
NERVE TERMINAL BLOCKER
RESERPINE
• Depletes catecholamines
• Dec sympathetic tone
• Inc parasymp tone • Inc gastric acid
• Dec BP°, Dec HR • Delayed onset
• Long duration • CNS depression
• Suicide
 	
GUANETHIDINE
•Depletes catecholamines
• Prevents release of catechols
• Major impairment of synapse
• Very potent
• Orthostatic hypotension
 	
GANGLIONIC BLOCKING AGENT
TRIMETHAPHAN
• Short acting
• IV drip
• Use for hypertensive emergency
	Very popular
	Good quality of life
	
	EFFECTS
	• Dec Angiotensin II
	• Inc Bradykinin
	• Dec PR – dec BP°
	• Large inc renin
	• NO reflex
	  tachycardia
	
	SIDE EFFECTS
	• Neutropenia
	• Proteinuria
	• Affects taste
	• Rash
	• Cough
	• Hepatotoxicity
	  (Captopril)
	
	TX
	Good for high-renin
	  hypertensives
	
	CONTRAINDICATED
	Bilateral renal
	  artery stenosis
	
	NO orthostatic
	hypotension, it
	does not interfere
	with sympathetics
	
	Proven to help reduce
	incidence of dilated
	cardiomyopathy
	and MI, 2° to
	hypertension
	
	Patient with
	hypertension and
	post-MI, good
	afterload reducer
		α METHYL DOPA
		(Aldomet®)
		• α_2 Agonist
		• Dec Symp output,
		  Dec CO, Dec HR,
		  Dec BP°
		• Minimal orthostatic
		  hypotension
		• Reduces baseline, but
		  still responds
		• Centrally acting
		
		SIDE EFFECTS
		• Sedation
		• Dry mouth
		• Na^+ / water retention
		
		CLONIDINE
		• An imidazole
		• Resembles
		  sympathomimetics
		• α_2 agonist
		  Dec sympath, Dec
		  HR (brady), Dec CO,
		  Dec PR, Dec BP°
		• Some α_1 – PNS
		  Inc BP° transient,
		  then dec BP°
		  after it redistributes in
		  CNS (α_2)
		NEW THEORY Does NOT
		  act through α_2 receptors
		• Acts through imidazole
		  receptors
		Clonidine displacing
		  substance binds and
		  removes clonidine from
		  imidazole receptors
		SIDE EFFECTS
		• Dry mouth
		• Sedation
		• Lethargy
		• Na^+/water retention
		Never discontinue
		suddenly – rebound
		hypertension

ATRIAL ARRHYTHMIA[72]	SINUS ARRHYTHMIA	SINUS TACHYCARDIA	SINUS BRADYCARDIA	SINUS BLOCK	SINUS ARREST	SICK SINUS SYNDROME
	Related to respiration	HR 100 – 150 b/min Normal ECG Anxiety, fever, and inc sympathetic	HR < 60 b/min	Impulse conduction blocked	Pause in cardiac rhythm	Combination of: sinus bradycardia, sinus arrest, and sinus block
	No Tx necessary	No Tx, goes away	**IX** 1. Block Vagus N. ATROPINE (MUSC receptor block) 2. Stim β receptor ISOPROTERENOL (β agonist) 3. Pacemaker	**IX** 1. IV ATROPINE 2. ISOPROTERENOL	**IX** 1. ATROPINE 2. ISOPROTERENOL 3. Pacemaker	**IX** 1. ATROPINE 2. ISOPROTERENOL 3. Pacemaker

Dec Phase 4 depolarization (Dec HR) Drug (ACh), Inc K^+ out or dec Na^+/Ca^{++} in

Inc Phase 4 depolarization (Inc HR) Catechol (NE), Dec K^+ out, Inc Na^+/Ca^{++} in

ATRIAL ARRHYTHMIA	PREMATURE ATRIAL CONTRACTION	PAROXYSMAL ATRIAL TACHYCARDIA	ATRIAL FLUTTER	ATRIAL FIBRILLATION	PARADOXICAL SUPRAVENTRICULAR TACHYCARDIA (PSVT)	JUNCTIONAL ARRHYTHMIA

	PAC
	Ectopic atrial foci
	• If near SA node, P wave is normal
	• If in lower atria, P wave is inverted
	
	℞
	QUINIDINE & PROCAINAMIDE or PROPRANOLOL
	
	Dec automaticity of ectopic foci
	Inc automaticity of SA node
		PAT
		Ectopic atrial focus because of disease or ischemia
		Reentry
		• Unidirection block
		• Slow conduction
		
		℞
		1. Inc vagal activity
		  a. Cardiac massage, Valsalva, rub eyes
		  b. Alpha agonists PHENYLEPHRINE METHOXAMINE
		  c. Anti AChE EDROPHONIUM
		2. Ca⁺⁺ blocker D.O.C. VERAPAMIL Dec AV conduct DILTIAZEM
		3. Na⁺ block QUINIDINE, PROCAINIMIDE
		4. Beta blockers PROPRANOLOL (last resort medication)
		5. DIGITALIS Dec conduct velocity
		6. Cardioversion if all drugs fail
			Not all impulses are transmitted to ventricle
			Ectopic focus
			Circus ring
			QRS normal
			P wave is patterned
			
			℞
			1. VERAPAMIL is drug of choice
			2. QUINIDINE
			3. PROCAINAMIDE
			4. DIGITALIS
			5. Cardioversion
			
			PHENYTOIN or K⁺ when flutter is induced by DIGITALIS
			
			ATROPINE can block vagomimetic action of DIGITALIS
				Multiple ectopic foci – Asynchronous
				Fractionation is roving circus entry
				P waves: No pattern
				
				DIGITALIS causes flutter to become fibrillation
				• Often reverts to SA node
				• If it does not, then Tx: ATROPINE to block vagomimetic effects of DIGITALIS
				
				℞
				1. VERAPAMIL
				2. QUINIDINE
				3. PROCAINAMIDE
				4. DIGITALIS
				5. Cardioversion
					QUINIDINE is vagolytic (antimuscarinic) and causes inc AV conduction
					
					Concealed conduction
					
					℞
					DIGITALIS
					Inc refractory time
					
					PARADOXICAL
					• with elevated atrial rate, not all impulses conduct through AV node
					• slowing down atrial rate may actually increase number of impulses through AV node, depolarizing ventricles
						AV node has taken over as pacemaker
						
						P wave is hidden, inverted, or follows QRS
						
						℞
						1. VERAPAMIL
						2. QUINIDINE & PROCAINAMIDE
						3. DIGITALIS
						4. Cardioversion

Goal is to Dec conduction impulse to protect ventricles

VENTRICULAR ARRHYTHMIA[73]	PREMATURE VENTRICULAR CONTRACTION	VENTRICULAR TACHYCARDIA	VENTRICULAR FIBRILLATION	2° AV BLOCK MOBITZ I	2° AV BLOCK MOBITZ II	3° AV BLOCK COMPLETE BLOCK
ECG	PVC Ectopic foci Extended QRS NO P wave Reversed T wave Inc RR interval delay normal QRS "compensatory pause" Bigeminy Trigeminy	6 Consecutive PVC HR 150 – 200 b/min Abnormal QRS If QRS patterned, it's from one focus 1. Ectopic focus 2. Reentry	Inc automaticity Latent pacemaker 1. Multiple foci 2. Reentry Can be caused by: CATECHOLAMINE, DIGITALIS or ischemia Ventricles do not contract	Progressive inc in PR interval until QRS misses Block is usually at AV node	Some P waves are conducted, some are not PR interval is fixed, does not change Block is below AV node	Atria and ventricles beat independently of each other PP interval same RR interval same PR interval changes
TREATMENT	LIDOCAINE Loading Dose: 50 – 100 mg IV bolus at rate of 20 – 50 mg/min (Not orally) May repeat in 5 min Then 52 mg/kg/min [Plasma] = 2 – 6 µg/ml Maintenance Dose 2 – 4 mg/min	1. LIDOCAINE 2. DISOPYRAMIDE	1. Cardiac Shock (Defibrillator) 2. LIDOCAINE 3. BRETYLIUM	1. ATROPINE (IV) 2. ISOPROTERENOL 3. Artificial pacemaker	1. ATROPINE (IV) 2. ISOPROTERENOL 3. Artificial pacemaker	1. ATROPINE (IV) 2. ISOPROTERENOL 3. Artificial pacemaker

1° AV BLOCK

Prolonged PR interval is fixed, (does not change)
Usually no problem, could be drug SE
Just discontinue drug

CARDIAC CONDITIONS	BUNDLE BRANCH BLOCK	WOLFF-PARKINSON-WHITE	EARLY AFTER DEPOLARIZATION	DELAYED AFTER DEPOLARIZATION	REENTRY
	Pathway blocked Widens QRS One of the bundle branches (Left or Right) is blocked	Accessory pathway Bundle of Kent has faster conduction to ventricles with NO AV node delay Widens QRS delta wave Can cause reentry through accessory path or through normal conducting tissue.	EAD Oscillation of plateau Caused by: 1. DIGITALIS toxicity (Inc Ca⁺⁺) 2. Hypoxia 3. Stretched myocard because of scarred tissue	DAD Train of oscillations after repolarization has occurred → depolarizes Can go to ventricular tachycardia Caused by: 1. DIGITALIS toxicity (Inc Ca⁺⁺) 2. MI 3. CATECHOLAMINE Excess	 Conduction caused by: 1. Orthograde conduction must be blocked 2. Retrograde impulse conducted slowly through block 3. Cells not refractory
TREATMENT	1. ISOPROTERENOL 2. PACEMAKER	1. QUINIDINE & PROCAINAMIDE 2. PROPRANOLOL	1. VERAPAMIL 2. DILITIAZEM	1. VERAPAMIL 2. DILITIAZEM	1. Converting the one-way block into a two-way block 2. Removing one-way block and inc conduction velocity in damaged tissue LIDOCAINE & PHENYTOIN
		Contraindicated: 1. DIGITALIS (Inc conduction velocity) 2. VERAPAMIL			

ANTIARRHYTH-MIC DRUGS	**IA** Na+ BLOCKERS – slows conduction (moderate dec phase 0) K+ block – prolongs repolarization (phase 3)	
	QUINIDINE [78]	**PROCAINAMIDE** [79]

QUINIDINE [78]

ORAL preferred IM painful
IV hypotension (α block)
– reflex inc HR
80% plasma protein bound
Hydroxylated in liver (20% excreted unchanged)

• Interacts w/ oral anticoags, causes bleeding
• Displaces Digoxin and Digitoxin – arrhythmia
• Vagolytic (atropine-like) effect – inc HR
• Blocks α Rec – inc HR
• inc automaticity SA node – reflex because dec BP°
(α block) – anticholinergic (vagolytic)

INC METABOLISM BY
PHENYTOIN and PHENOBARBITAL

MECH OF ANTIARRHYTHMIC ACTION
blocks Na+ channels • dec responsiveness
• dv/dt dec conduction velocity
A. Reentry: dec Phase O
• Diseased tissue converts uni- to bi- directional
block by dec conduction velocity

B. Ectopic focus:
1. dec Phase 4 Depol of focus, dec automaticity
2. dec conduction velocity phase 0, low safety
factor

ECG
• inc PR interval
• inc ERP of His-Purkinje system
(not AV node – Ca++ response)
• inc QT = inc APD, blocks K+ channels phase 3
• widens QRS

TOXICITY
[QUIN]$_{plasma}$ > 5 mg/ml, [K+] > 5 mM
QRS widens > 30% – can precipitate arrhythmia
Quinidine Syncope: Light-headed
Torsade de pointes: disorganized V-tachycardia
Antimuscarinic: inc conduction thru AV node
and an inc SA rate (vagolytic) – paroxysmal inc HR

CONCEALED CONDUCTION
• dec number of atrial impulses
• dec refractory period of AV node
• lets more impulses go thru • inc HR (paroxysmal)
• Give Digitalis before
Sick Sinus Synd: QUIN marked dec pacemaker
activity

SIDE EFFECTS
GI: nausea, vomiting, diarrhea
CINCHONISM: headache, dizziness, tinnitus

USE
1° – supravent arrhythmias: PAC, PAT, A. Flut/Fib,
WPW, Interatrial and AV node reentry
2° – ventricular arrhythmia, PVC, vent. tachycardia

PROCAINAMIDE [79]

ORAL chronic Tx
IV
Life threatening situations
(arrhyth) (monitor BP° fall)
• 100 mg/15 min
• conc. 3 –10 µg/ml
IV infusion
20% Plasma protein bnd
Metab in liver to NAPA –
also antiarrhythmic

CARDIAC EFFECTS
• same as QUINIDINE
except weaker:
• vagolytic
• α blocking

ECG
same as QUIN
Weak Atropine-like
effect, NO α block

TOXICITY
1. SLE-like Syndrome
• Arthritis
• Arthralgia
• Pericarditis
• Peritonitis
2. Other
• Nausea, diarrhea
• Agranulocytosis →
2° infections

CNS
• Depression
• Hallucination

USE
1° – same as QUIN
• 2nd choice after
LIDOCAINE for vent
arrhyth due to MI
2° – same as QUIN

NO / little paradoxical
inc HR
Better (-) inotropic

SIDE EFFECTS
• Dec peripheral
resistance
– hypotension

IA	IB	Na⁺ BLOCKERS – slow conduction

IB — Na⁺ BLOCKERS – slow conduction
Inc K⁺ permeability – shorten repolarization

DISOPYRAMIDE [80]	LIDOCAINE [81]	PHENYTOIN [82]
USA - oral only 30% plasma protein bound Metabolized in liver CARDIAC same as QUIN ECG same as QUIN OTHER EFFECTS Much greater antimuscarinic than Quinidine (vagolytic) Parox inc Vent HR – Digitalis must be given before atrial flutter or fibrillation develops NO α block Weak Ca⁺⁺ channel block TOXICITY • Arrhythmia • Heart failure • Urinary retention • Dry mouth • Blurred vision • Constipation • Aggravates glaucoma USE Ventricular tachycardia if LIDOCAINE fails	ORAL NOT effective – extensively metabolized IM OK IV Preferred Inject 100 mg loading dose Infuse 52 µg/kg/min 10 – 60% protein bound CARDIAC EFFECTS NOT as pronounced an effect on Na⁺ channels as the group IA drugs • Cond vel, small dec • dec Phase 3 repolarization by opening K⁺ channels • net dec APD NO EFFECT AVN or HR ECG NO noticeable change Ventricular muscle is much more sensitive – LIDO works better against V arrhythmias SIDE EFFECTS (Like any local anesthesia) • Convulsions • Hearing & speech problems • Nausea of central origin USE Arrhyth assoc with Depol 1° Vent tachycardia during MI or cardiac surgery PVC (ischemic) 2° Digitalis induced ventricle arrhythmias [NOT effective against normal polarized tissue arrhythmias (A. flutter)]	ORAL absorbed slowly IV Divided doses to prevent collapse Infusion – causes phlebitis 90% plasma protein bound METAB Hydroxylated Na⁺ channel block Some Ca⁺⁺ blocking Dec symp activity in the CNS DIGITALIS TOXICITY – inc symp stimulation 1. Delay after depol that reaches threshold "trigger arrhythmia" 2. Inc symp activity in CNS DIG Tox Tx: PHENYTOIN – some Ca⁺⁺ block (VERAPAMIL) METABOLISM 1. Decreased by • DICUMAROL (Coumadin) (oral anticoagulant) • ISONIAZID (anti TB drug) 2. Increased by PHENOBARB TOXICITY CNS: • Depression • Ataxia • Vertigo GI: • Anorexia • Vomiting Hypersensitive • Stevens-Johnson • Erythema multiforme Hyperglycemia • dec insulin secretion Gingival hyperplasia • alters collagen Megaloblastic anemia • alters folate metabolism USE • Digitalis-induced ventricle arrhythmias • Anticonvulsant

TOCAINIDE, MEXILETINE [83]

Congeners of LIDOCAINE
ORAL
  resistant to metabolism first pass effect
CARDIAC EFFECTS
  same as Lidocaine
TOXICITY
  TOCAINIDE produces serious, sometimes fatal hematological disorders

PHENYTOIN and LIDOCAINE

Can remove unidirectional blocks by improving conduction velocity in damaged areas

ANTIARRHYTH- MIC DRUGS	IC [84] ENCAINIDE FLECAINIDE LORCAINIDE	II BETA BLOCK PROPRANOLOL [85]	III LONGER REPOLARIZATION	
			AMIODARONE [86]	BRETYLIUM [87]
ADMINISTRATION	Very potent Dec dv/dt Marked dec phase 0 Dec conduction velocity • Na+ blocker NO effect on repolarization	ORAL excellent absorption • inc dose because of first pass effect IV can use lower dose 90% plasma protein bound	Orally $T_{1/2}$ 13 – 103 days, Load 15 – 30 days, Limited use, too slow and toxic Inc APD (inc QT)	IM or IV Short term emergency NOT metabolized Excreted unchanged $T_{1/2}$ = 9 hrs
MODE OF ACTION		CARDIAC EFFECT β blocker • dec symp stim • inhib arrhythmia Very high conc – local anesthetic Plasma [] = 100 – 300 ng/ml Dec arrhythmia • dec automaticity in SA node and in ectopic foci • dec cond velocity in AV node At high plasma [ ] 1000 ng/ml – dec dv/dt rate of rise of phase 0 Inc PR interval	Blocks K+ channels, delays repolarization Inc ERP = PR interval at AV node Dec sinus rate – β block, also has α block (Tx: Angina in Europe) • α & β block • dec O_2 demand • dec symp activity	Blocks K+ channels prolongs repolarization Inc APD and inc ERP to normal – Ischemia Inc PR interval • inc QT • dec sinus rate ISCHEMIA Vent–Purkinje • dec APD • dec ERP • gets reversed by drug
	USE Wolff- Parkinson- White Syndrome • suppresses accessory pathway • C.A.S.T. excessive		Ca++ channel block vasodilation of coronary arteries Some Na+ blocking properties • dv/dt • dec conduction velocity in diseased cells	Only in ventricles, NOT atria SIDE EFFECT • Concentrate in adrenerg nerve terminal • initially causes release NE • later it prevents release
TOXICITY		TOXICITY cardiovascular • dec HR • dec BP° • dec contractility SIDE EFFECT • Asthmatic – lethal bronchoconstriction • Aminophylline as an antidote	SIDE EFFECT Bradycardia, heart block, fatal lung fibrosis, hepatic necrosis, altered thyroid function (iodine in the drug) corneal deposit, skin pigmentation	TOXICITY Hypotension
USE		USE 1° Wolff-Parkinson-White Syndrome 2° Prophylaxis of atrial and ventricular post-infarction tachyarrhythmia Treat sympathetic arrhythmia	USE NOT popular U.S. (Europe: angina and Wolff-Parkinson-White Syndrome)	USE Emergency setting, when LIDOCAINE and electric shock fail to terminate vent fibrillation

IV Ca++ CHANNEL BLOCKERS

MECHANISM Slow Ca++ channel blocker

ANGINA 1. Relax coronary arteries and arterioles in ischemic and normal heart
  • Inhibit coronary art spasm, inc coronary blood flow, inc O_2 delivery
2. Relax systemic arteries • dec BP° • dec afterload, dec O_2 demand

ARRHYTHMIA dec conduction in AV node • dec number of impulses delivered to ventricle during Paroxysmal Supravent Tachycardia

VERAPAMIL[88]	NIFEDIPINE [89] (Procardia®)	DILTIAZEM [90]
Oral: Angina: Prinzmetal's, chronic stable, unstable † IV: Arrhythmia † († U.S. only) • 90% absorb • Onset < 30 min • Peak 5 hr • 90% protein bound • Metab liver =15% bioavail • Excreted: urine	Oral: Angina: Prinzmetal's, chronic stable IV: Arrhythmia , Sublingual: • 90% absorb • Peak 1– 2 hr • Onset < 20 min (3 min Subl) • 90% prt bnd • Metab liver = 65% bioavail • Excreted: urine	Oral: Angina: Prinzmetal's, chronic stable IV: Arrhythmia • 90% absorb • Onset < 30 min • Peak 30 min • 80% protein bound • Metab liver < 20% bioavail • Excreted: feces
	Calcium Channel Inhibition	
+++	+++	+++
	Dec AV Nodal Conduction (antiarrhythmic)	
++++	+/-	+++
	Smooth Muscle Relaxing Coronary Art	
+++	++++	+++
	Systemic Art	
+++	++++	+++
	Decrease in Blood Pressure	
Modest	Significant	Modest
	Veins	
0	0	0
	Heart Rate Direct Effect	
Small dec	Large dec	Small dec
	Heart Rate Reflex Effect	
Small dec	Large inc	Small dec
	Heart Rate Net Effect	
Little change	Small inc	Little change
	Negative Inotropy	
++	+	++

USE (Verapamil) reentrant supravent arrhyth, reduce vent rate in atrial fib and atrial flutter , Wolff-Parkinson-White, tachyarrhythmia
They DO NOT reduce ventricle ectopic foci (All the other antiarrhythmics do)
TOXICITY 1. hypotension 2. myocardial depression 3. heart failure 4. dizziness 5. flushing 6. bradycardia

TYPES OF ANGINA

1. STABLE: Brief pain 3 - 5 min after exertion
2. PROGRESSIVE: Stable after a few months • becomes more frequent and severe
3. DECUBITUS: Pain at rest and reclined position
4. NOCTURNAL: During sleep
5. UNSTABLE: Angina changes intensity
6. PRINZHEIMER'S: Pain at rest, not exercise or emotional stress,
    ST segment is elevated • may be NO coronary artery disease
      (all other angina's lower ST segment)
    Coronary artery spasms • dec flow
                              • dec O_2 supply (not an increase O_2 demand)

CAUSES OF ANGINA

Anatomic: 90% lesions • Atherosclerosis
Functional: Aortic stenosis • obstruct flow, dec O_2 supply, thyrotoxicosis
                              • inc O_2 demand and tachycardia
Angina attacks: Depress ST segment, changes T wave, then goes back to normal
  (reversible)

	Nitrates	β Blocker	Combined
BP°	dec BP°	dec BP°	dec BP°
Contractility	inc (reflex)	dec (direct)	——
HR	inc (reflex)	dec (direct)	——
EDV	dec EDV	inc EDV	——

ANTI ANGINAL DRUGS	NITRATES and NITRITES	β BLOCKERS	Ca++ BLOCK-ERS
EXAMPLE	**NITROGLYCERIN** [91]	**PROPRANOLOL**[92]	**VERAPAMIL** [93]
ADMINISTRATION	Sublingual, transdermal Short acting • NITROGLYCERIN • AMYL NITRITE • ISOSORBIDE DINITRATE Long acting – hours • NITROGLYCERIN • ISOSORBIDE DINITRATE • PENTAERYTHRITOL TETRANITRATE • ERYTHRITYL TETRANITRATE For long lasting oral effect – inc dose to get by first pass Vasodilate – dec afterload Venodilate – dec preload DILATORY EFFECT Vein > large arteries > arterioles • Perfuses ischemic areas TX Angina SIDE EFFECTS • Hypotension • Dizziness • Weakness • Spastic angina • Headache (meningeal vessels dilate) • Flushing • MHb (use in C=N poisoning)	Dec sympathetics • dec HR • dec BP° • dec contractility • inc exercise tolerance • dec O_2 demand TX Stable and unstable angina SIDE EFFECTS 1. Congestive heart failure with prolonged use • dec CO • reflex renal accum Na^+, H_2O • leads to edema and CHF 2. Bradycardia • dec SA rate 3. Heart block • dec conduction CONTRAINDICATED WITH 1. Asthmatics • Inhibits bronchodilation 2. Hypoglycemics • inhibits recovery from hypo-glycemia	Dec Ca++ to smooth muscle • inhibits contraction • prevents phosphoryla-tion of myosin Promotes relaxation and dilation

DISOPYRAMIDE [94]
Dilatory effect • 1° on arterioles • Perfuse all tissue equally "Coronary Steal" • NOT for angina Dec PLT aggregation • Prophylactic for atherosclerosis

ANTI-COAGULANTS	DIRECT ANTICOAGULANT [95]	INDIRECT ANTICOAGULANT [96]	ANTITHROMBOTIC [97]	THROMBOLYTIC [98]
DRUGS	HEPARIN (immediate effect) EDTA SODIUM CITRATE	DICUMAROL WARFARIN	DIPYRIDAMOLE ASPIRIN	STREPTOKINASE UROKINASE TISSUE PLASMINOGEN ACTIVATOR (TPA)

ADMINISTRATION	HEPARIN (only one approved)
	Intravenous
	• Large negative molecule
	• Does NOT cross membranes
	• Pregnant women can take it
	Oral – poorly absorbed
	IM – hematoma
		DICUMAROL
		• Absorption is too erratic
		
		WARFARIN
		ORAL
		Completely absorbed
		Lipid soluble
		  • crosses membranes
		NOT for pregnant women
		Delay effect 8 – 12 hr
		99% albumin-bound
		  • can be displaced
			• Suppresses PLT function
			
			ASPIRIN
			• Inhibit cyclooxygenase
			• Inhibit synthesis thromboxane A2
			
			DIPYRIDAMOLE
			• Unknown mechanism
			• Does NOT work alone
			• Used with WARFARIN
				IV or intracoronary
				Dissolves both venous and arterial clots
				
				TPA
				• High affinity keeps it local
				• Activates plasminogen into plasmin:
				1. Degrade clotting factors
				2. Degrade adhesive proteins

MECHANISM	**MECH** Enhances Antithrombin III
	ATIII – inactivates Factors II, IX, XIII and Kallikrein
	Saturates liver enzymes that break it down
	• 0° kinetics • inc dose • inc T₁/₂
	SIDE EFFECTS (high dose)
	– Depletes ATIII – massive clot formations • hemorrhage
	Tx for high dose:
	  1. Dec dose
	  2. PROTAMINE SULFATE
	    • inhibits heparin
	    • also an anticoag
	– Thrombocytopenia
	Rx venous thrombi (red) – acts on fibrin – contracts blood clot
		MECH
		Inhibits Vit K dependent
		1. Synthesis II, VII, IX, X
		2. Epoxide Vit K reductase
		3. Synthesis of prothrombin
		
		WARFARIN TOXICITY
		Tx – antidote: Vitamin K
		
		Rx
		Venous thrombi (red) acts on fibrin
			Rx Arterial thrombi (white) acts on platelets	STREPTOKINASE
				UROKINASE
				  • both disseminate
				
				SIDE EFFECT
				  • may cause widespread hemorrhaging
				
				All three have equal effectiveness and mortality

STAGES OF CLOT FORMATION

1. PLATELET ADHESION: Blood vessel breaks, collagen exposed, platelets adhere
   Three requirements:
   1. Free amino groups on collagen
   2. Fibrinogen
   3. von Willebrand's Factor VIIIR

2. PLATELET AGGREGATION: Platelets release granules
   1. Adhesion factor – chemotaxis
   2. Thromboxane A2 – pseudopodia form
   3. Serotonin – constricts blood vessel

3. COAGULATION:
   1. Fibrin – traps RBCs, stops flow
   2. Thrombin – stabilizes plug

4. REPAIR: After repaired, plasmin degrades fibrin

CASCADE
Important Points: Hageman Factor XII initiates,
Intrinsic pathway takes minutes, extrinsic takes seconds, both are needed

THROMBI
1. Arterial thrombi (white) – predominantly platelets   Tx: antithrombotics
2. Venous thrombi (red) – predominantly fibrin   Tx: anticoagulants

DIURETICS	OSMOTIC [99]	CARBONIC [100] ANHYDRASE INHIBITORS	THIAZIDES [101] (Ca^{++} Sparing)
DRUGS	UREA ISOSORBIDE MANNITOL	ACETAZOLAMIDE	CHLOROTHIAZIDE HYDROCHLOROTHIAZIDE

ADMINISTR.
 	
MECHANISM
 	
USE
 	
1° EFFECT
dec ECF
	Oral : poorly
	    absorbed
	IV: preferred, water
	  soluble, uncharged
	NOT metabolized
	Filtered renal
	• inc urine flow
	• only slight inc
	  NaCl excreted
	• slight inc K$^+$ excreted
	PCT 70% Na$^+$
	  reabsorbed
	ISOSORBIDE
	• dec intraocular P°
	• Acute cases
	
	MANNITOL
	Prevents renal
	  failure during:
	• cardiovasc surgery
	• trauma
	• transfusion
	  reactions
	dec CSF
	dec intraocular P°
	Toxic: kidney injury
	
	SIDE EFFECT
	•Expands ECF, risky
	  with heart patient
	  (inc plasma K$^+$)
	• Nausea • Vomiting
	• Headache
		Oral: well
		    absorbed
		Rapid onset
		< 30 min
		Penetrates CNS
		Sulfamyl group
		  (so is secreted)
		NOT metabolized
		Rapid renal
		  excretion
		• filtration
		• secreted
		MECH
		• Block formation
		  of H ions
		• PCT and DCT
		• inc NaHCO$_3$
		  excretion
		1. Loss bicarb
		  • metab acidosis
		2. inc Na$^+$ excreted
		  inc K$^+$ excreted
		  inc urine vol
		3. slight Ca^{++} excret-
		  ion, insignificant
		Tolerance
		  3 – 4 days
		USE
		• Diuretic
		• Epilepsy
		• Glaucoma
		• Hyper &
		  hypokalemic
		  paralysis
		• Alkalinize urine
		• Acute mountain
		  sickness
		SIDE EFFECTS
		• Somnolence
		• Fatigue
		• Paresthesia
			Oral: absorbed
			LIMITED PENETRATION
			  INTO CNS – so not used
			  for epileptics or
			  intraocular P°
			Rapid clearance
			  Sulfamyl group – secreted
			Dec Bld Vol & PR, Dec BP°
			
			MECH
			• Block NaCl transport
			  (in early DCT)
			• weak Carb Anhyd
			  inhibitor (sulfamyl
			  group property)
			• inc Na$^+$ excretion
			• inc K$^+$ excretion
			• dec Ca^{++} excretion
			• not effect HCO$_3$ =
			• Site: PCT
			
			HYDROCHLOROTHIAZIDE
			• Short acting
			• 70% absorbed
			• Rapid onset
			• Peak 2 – 4 hrs
			• T$_{1/2}$ = 8 – 10 hrs
			• PCT: filtered & secreted
			
			CHLOROTHIAZIDE
			• Long acting
			• 20% absorbed
			• Slow onset
			• T$_{1/2}$ = 48 hrs
			USE
			• Antihypertensive
			• Edema
			• Diabetes I (ADH resistant)
			• Hypercalciuria
			• Ca^{++} stones
			SIDE EFFECTS
			• Hyperuricemia
			• Hypokalemia (K$^+$ loss)
			• Hyperglycemia
			• Hypochloremic
			  alkalosis (H$^+$ & Cl$^-$ loss)
			• Mg^{++} loss
			• Inc TAG (plasma)

CARBONIC ANHYDRASE (CA)

$$H_2O + CO_2$$
$$\uparrow CA$$
$$H_2CO_3^-$$
$$\uparrow$$
$$HCO_3^-$$
$$\uparrow$$
$$NaHCO_3$$

$$CO_2 + H_2O \overset{CA}{\longleftrightarrow} H_2CO_3^-$$

$$H^+ \qquad H^+ \qquad HCO_3^= \rightarrow NaHCO_3$$
$$Na^+ \rightarrow Na^+$$

Inhibit CA – No H ion out
           – inc excretion of Na$^+$, HCO$_3$=, H$_2$O

LOOP DIURETICS [102]	K⁺ SPARING [103]
ETHACRYNIC ACID FUROSEMIDE	TRIAMTERENE AMILORIDE SPIRONOLACTONE

FUROSEMIDE
(Bumetanide is similar)

Oral: well absorbed

Penetrates CNS

Large renal clearance

Sulfamyl group
 • secreted
 • weak CA inhibitor

Rapid onset

Short duration 4 – 6 hrs

MECH
 • Blocks Na⁺, K⁺, Cl⁻ cotransport
   (in ascending loop of Henle)
 • PCT – weak CA inhibitor
      – blocks Na⁺ transport
 • DCT – dec Ca⁺⁺ reabsorption
 • Direct smooth muscle relaxer
 • inc NaCl excretion
 • inc K⁺ excretion (Na⁺ and K⁺ excretion
   greatest in loop diuretics)
 • some inc Ca⁺⁺ excretion

SIDE EFFECTS
 • Hyperuricemia
 • Hypokalemia
 • Hyponatremia
 • Hyperglycemia
 • Hypochloremic alkalosis
 • Hearing deficit

ETHACRYNIC ACID
ORAL Good absorption

Rapid excretion – PCT
 • inc NaCl excretion
 • inc K⁺ excretion
 • inc Ca⁺⁺ excretion
   (greater than FUROSEMIDE)

SIDE EFFECTS
 • Hyperuricemia
 • Hypokalemia
 • Hyponatremia
 • Hyperglycemia
 • Hypochloremic alkalosis
   (like FUROSEMIDE)
 • Diarrhea (severe)

> Both can be used in Tx of:
> • Acute pulmonary edema
> • Hypertension

SPIRONOLACTONE
 • Resembles aldosterone
 • Competitive inhibitor
 • Slow onset   •Long duration
 • Liver metabolites – many

MECH
 • inc Na⁺ excreted • K⁺ retained • weak diuretic

USE
 • 1° Aldosteronism
 • with THIAZIDE drugs to dec K⁺ loss
 • with LOOP DIURETICS in cirrhosis patients

SIDE EFFECTS
 • Gynecomastia • Menstrual changes
 • Hyperkalemia

TRIAMTERENE
 • Resembles folic acid • Rapid onset – 2 hr
 • NOT metabolized
 • Excreted unchanged – urine

MECH
 • Block Na⁺, K⁺ excretion (in DCT)
 • dec H excretion • weak diuretic
 • some HCO₃⁻ excreted • NaCl excreted

USES
 • with other diuretics, to dec K⁺ loss
 • NOT with cirrhotic patients

SIDE EFFECTS
 • Hyperkalemia, vomiting, dizziness

AMILORIDE
 • Pyrazine ring • One dose / day
 • Rapid onset • Excreted unchanged
 • NOT metabolized

MECH • dec Na⁺ reabsorption
        • weak diuretic

USE • NOT for initial therapy
      • Only if inc K⁺ loss

SIDE EFFECTS
 • Shock • Weakness, flaccid paralysis
 • Bradycardia, change in ECG

CONTRAINDICATED
 1. Renal insufficiency
 2. Diabetic neuropathy
 3. Anuria
 4. Do NOT give K⁺ supplement

3 NERVOUS SYSTEM

CNS STIMULANTS	PSYCHOMOTOR [141] STIMULANTS	METHYLXANTHINE [142]
	AMPHETAMINE (Benzedrine®) METHYLPHENIDATE (Ritalin®) – D.O.C. •Releases monoamines (NE, 5H-T...) • Inhibits reuptake USE • Hyperkinetic • Attention Deficit Syndrome • Narcolepsy SIDE EFFECTS • Dizziness • Tremor • Irritability • Addictive • Coma • Convulsions FENFLURAMINE • Use for obesity • Generally NOT therapeutic	1. CAFFEINE – Coffee, Cola 2. THEOPHYLLINE – Chocolate, limited CNS stimulant 3. THEOBROMINE – Tea, Less CNS stim CNS Stimulants: CAFFEINE > THEOPHYLLINE > THEOBROMINE Diuresis Stimulation of heart Related structurally to uric acid Does NOT make gout worse Fits well in DNA Caffeine may be mutagenic USES 1. Status Epilepticus • AMINOPHYLLINE (Theophylline + Ethylendiame) 2. Bronchodilation 3. Reduces fatigue • Inc muscle work capacity EFFECTS 1. Constricts cerebral vessels 2. Dilates peripheral vessels (Coronary vessels) 3. Inc cardiac output 4. Diuresis SIDE EFFECTS 1. Impairment of precise motor and mental function 2. Nervousness 3. Insomnia 4. Delirium 5. Tremors 6. Rebound headache with withdrawal 7. Irritable MECHANISM OF ACTION 1. Inc in intracellular Ca^{++} at high doses 2. Inhibits phosphodiesterase • Inc cAMP 3. Binds Ca^{++} channels / GABA receptors • Dec Cl^- permeability 4. Adenosine receptors in brain competitively blocked (Xanthine) CAFFEINE competes with BENZODIAZEPINES – get anxiety

SLEEP DISORDERS	EXCESSIVE SOMNOLENCE	Δ SLEEP/WAKE CYCLE
NORMAL SLEEP 4 Stages Awake – REM. . . 4 Later at night – more 2 Longer REM as night progresses 50% in Stage 2 25% in REM Remainder in stages 3 – 4 **REM** 1. Move toward α 2. Active inhibition of skeletal muscles 3. Rapid Eye Movement 4. Dream recall best 5. Dreaming 6. Inc BP° and HR 7. Inc GH release 8. Deprive REM • Rebound REM • Nightmares Children • More Stage 4 Elderly • Little Stage 3 • NO Stage 4 • Little REM **SLEEP DISORDERS** 1. Disorder initiating & maintaining sleep (DIMS= insomnia) 2. Hypersomnia – excess somnolence 3. Sleep/Wake cycle Δ 4. Parasomnias	During Day During Night 1. **NARCOLEPSY** [104] • Irresistible urge to sleep 1 – 15 min Three symptoms may be present: a. Cataplexy – loss of muscle tone b. Sleep paralysis c. Hypnagogic hallucination Sudden attack REM – Very Short REM High Assoc HLA–DR2 **TX** CNS stimulations & inhibition of REM sleep *AMPHETAMINE *METHYLAMPHETAMINE *PROPRANOLOL *METHYLPHENIDATE *PHENELZINE (MAO inhibitor) *TCA –Tx 3 symptoms 2. **SLEEP APNEA** [105] > 10 sec • Fluctuates blood gases • Many types • Obstructive apnea • Loud snoring • NO real drug Tx • Positive nasal air P° • Surgical intervention	Jet lag Work shift Δ **PARASOMNIAS** [106] Occur at night NOT by Sleep/Wake mechanism 1. **SLEEP WALK** 6 – 12 yr olds • During slow-wave sleep • NOT a dream being enacted • Resist walking • NOT dangerous If need Tx: Use Benzodiazepine: *DIAZEPAM (Valium®) *FLURAZEPAM • Inhibits Stage 4 • Inc sedation 2. **SLEEP TERRORS** • 1° children • NOT a nightmare • Sit up screaming • Late Stage 3/4 • Symp discharge • Tx if needed *Benzodiazepine

INSOMNIA (DIMS) [107]

TYPES
1. Psychophysiologic
   a. Transient – most common – stress
   b. Persistent
2. Psychiatric Disorders
3. Drugs and alcohol
4. Nocturnal myoclonus – elderly
5. Respiratory sleep impairment
6. Medications

NONPHARMACOLOGICAL TREATMENT
1. Dec caffeine, alcohol or drugs
2. Regular sleep hours
3. Reduce stress

SEDATIVES / HYPNOTICS
SEDATIVE: Calming effect with no effect on motor activity or cognitive activity
HYPNOTIC: Induces state resembling sleep
Sed – Hyp – Coma – Death

INSOMNIA (DIMS) [107]

BARBITURATES
Na+ salt, weak acid
Well absorbed
BARBITURIC ACID = 2,4,6-
    trioxohexahydropyrimidine
Metabolized – liver microsomal enzymes
    Mixed function oxidases
Inc polarity – excretion

TWO CLASSES
1. ANESTHETICS (Sulf)
   • Rapid Onset (IV) – short duration
     *THIOPENTAL *METHOHEXITAL [108]
   • Taken up quickly into brain
   • Redistributes to fat stores
   • Metabolized slowly
2. SEDATIVE/ HYPNOTICS (Oxy)
   • Less lipid soluble *PHENOBARBITAL
     *AMOBARBITAL *SECOBARBITAL[109]
     *PENTABARBITAL
   • Identical to THIOPENTAL, except S is
     replaced by O
   • More evenly distributed
   • Rely on metab for termination
   • Longer duration

PHARMACOLOGY
   • General depressants
   • Inhibit heart & autonomic ganglia

MECHANISM OF ACTION
   • Unclear, NO receptor, NO antidote
   • Affects synapses
   • Facilitates GABA effects (-)
     (Inhibitor NT)
     Opens up Cl⁻ channels

BARBITURATE EFFECT ON SLEEP
   • Dec latency • Inc duration • Suppress
     REM by 25% • Some dec in Stage 4
   • Within a week recover REM
Respiratory depressant
     Inhibits CO_2 receptors in the CNS
CardioVasc • Only toxic dose • Dec BP°
T° – hypothermic
NOT analgesic – Hyper-response to pain

OD ACUTE TOXICITY
1. Mild – Unconscious, pain response
2. Deep – Less corneal reflex
3. Severe – Dec BP, HR, CO; NO pain,
   NO Tx for BARB toxicity • Do NOT give
   stimulant • Supportive therapy
Highly addictive
Gradual withdrawal from drug

CHRONIC TOXICITY – Not frequent
1. Allergic reaction – local, eyelids swell
   rash, exfoliative dermatitis
2. Extremes of age – agitate, delirium
3. Porphyria – porphyrins synth by liver
   Excess porph – behavior Δ, GI Δ

CHLORAL HYDRATE [110]
Reduced in many tissues (esp RBC) to
   active metab TRICHLORETHANOL
   (wide use Peds & Geriatric Med/Dent)
Less REM Inhibition
Easier sedative effect
Alcohol accentuates ALL CNS depressors,
   Esp with CHLORAL HYDRATE
GI DISTURBANCES
   • Pediatrics
   • Give Antihist/Antiemetic agent
     HYDROXYZINE, DRAMAMINE®

ANTIHISTAMINES [111]
Sedation/Hypnosis as side effects
*DIPHENHYDRAMINE (OTC)
   antimuscarinic (anticholinergic) SE
*DOXYLAMINE
   • NO Antichol side effect
Use: Mild, moderate insomnia Tx
Idiosyncratic response – Children
*GLUTETHIMIDE – like a BARB
   • Abused, combined with cocaine

BENZODIAZEPINES [112] (Inc GABA effects)
Short: minor suppression of REM sleep
Long acting BDZ – NO REM suppression
Selective suppress Stage 4 – NO rebound
NO signif induct hepatic microsome enz
Far LESS ADDICTIVE
*CHLORODIAZEPOXIDE
   (alcohol withdrawal)
*DIAZEPAM (Valium®)
*FLURAZEPAM • 30 mg, $T_{1/2}$ = 60 hr
                • Sedation/Hypnosis next
                  day, 3 metabolites
*TEMAZEPAM • T = 5 – 10 hr (night)
*TRIAZOLAM • $T_{1/2}$ = 4 hr, potent,
                but may not be kept
                asleep entire night,
                Rebound insomnia
*LORAZEPAM • Intermediate acting
                • Contraindicated:
                  Narrow Angle Glaucoma

ANTI DEPRESSANT	TRICYCLIC ANTIDEPRESSANTS [113]	MAO INHIBITORS [114]	
		HYDRAZIDE	NONHYDRAZIDE
	IMIPRAMINE (Triavil®) 3° amine AMITRIPTYLINE (Elavil®) 3° amine DESIPRAMINE – 2° amine, metabolite of Imipramine	PHENELZINE ISOCARBOXAZID	TRANYLCYPRO-MINE

	1° INDICATION
	1. Major depressive episodes
	2. Enuresis (bed wetting)
	   Anticholinergic
	
	D.O.C. for depression
	MECH Blocks 5-HT and NE
	   Postsynaptic reuptake
	   • Inc mood
	SIDE EFFECTS
	1. Anticholinergic (atropine-like)
	   • tachycardia, blurred vision, dry mouth, memory loss, urinary retention
	2. Cardiovascular • tachycardia
	   • orthostatic hypotension
	3. Hand tremors
	4. Mild headache
	5. Sedation, weakness
	   Increases Phase 4 sleep
	PHARMACOKINETICS
	   • highly lipid soluble, slowly absorbed, slow onset – weeks, high volume distribution, 1st pass metabolism, high plasma protein binding, displaced by ASPIRIN, $T_{1/2}$ = 12 hr
	INTERACTIONS
	1. Antipsychotics • Δ metabolism
	2. GUANETHIDINE uptake inhibited at the neuron
	   (Dec effect of Guanethidine)
	DOSE Determined Empirically
	OD
	1. Severe 5. Seizures
	   Hypotension or 6. Coma
	2. Hypertension 7. Convulsion
	3. Arrhythmia 8. Death
	4. Hyperpyrexia
	Treat OD
	a. PHYSOSTIGMINE • Inc ACh
	b. DIAZEPAM (Valium®)
	   • counter Anti ACh
	WITHDRAWAL should be gradual
	   • Too abruptly = Nausea, dizziness, sweat, headaches, salivate
		Irreversible
		
		INDICATIONS
		1. Phobic anxiety
		2. Post Traumatic Stress
		3. Bulimia
		4. Narcolepsy
		5. Depression (Same for TCA, if TCAs fail)
		
		MECHANISM
		Block oxidative deamination of monoamines (catecholamines, indoles)
		Inhibits monoamine degradation
		   Inc mood
		Inc availability of neurotransmitter
		   • Enhances effect on β receptor
		   • Delayed onset
		
		SIDE EFFECTS
		1. Tremors
		2. Agitation
		3. Insomnia
		4. Orthostatic hypotension
		5. Hypertensive uresis
		   • w/ exogenous monoamines
		   • exaggerates effects of tyramine in diet
		6. Profound release of histamine
		Tx Side Effect: PHENTOLAMINE
		   • Adrenergic blocker
		
		PHARMACOKINETICS
		   • Orally
		   • Rapid distribution
		   • HYDRAZINES are acetylated
		   • 75% MAO inhibition for effect
		
		DRUG INTERACTION
		1. TCAs & MAOIs – NEVER use together
		2. TCAs & Alcohol or BARBs
		   • Central depression
			Reversible

2nd GENERATION ANTIDEPRESSANT DRUGS

AMOXAPINE – Blocks 5-HT and NE reuptake [115]
MAPROTILINE – Blocks NE reuptake
TRAZODONE – Blocks 5-HT and α_2 receptors
MIANSERIN – Blocks α_2, Hist, and 5-HT
    postsynaptic receptors
ALPRAZOLAM – Antianxiety, short acting
BUPROPION – Inhibits DA reuptake

PYSCHOMOTOR STIMULATION [116]
AMPHETAMINE
DEXTRA AMPHETAMINE
    – Sympathomimetic
USE Elderly
NOT effective antidepressants

LITHIUM [117]
 Inc reuptake of NE and 5-HT
    – Dec mood
USE
 Manic episodes

CONTRAINDICATED
 – Renal failure

ELECTROCONVULSIVE THERAPY
 ECT – last resort

EFFECTIVE
 Noncompliant, depressed,
 90% remission rate

FLUOXETINE (Prozac®) [118]
• New drug
• 5-HT uptake inhibitor
• Some NE uptake inhibition
• 95% protein bound
• Metabolized by liver
• Excreted by kidney
SIDE EFFECTS
 Rash, urticaria, vasculitis, fever,
 leukocytosis, arthralgia, edema,
 resp distress, lymphadenopathy,
 headache, dizziness, nausea, GI
PRECAUTION
 Anxiety, insomnia, dec weight and
 appetite, mania, seizures, suicide

DEPRESSION

BIOCHEMISTRY
    1. Decrease in NE, 5-HT, and/or DA
    2. Increase in β receptors

CAUSES
    1. RESERPINE – depletes catecholamines
    2. α METHYL PARA TYROSINE – tyrosine hydroxylase inhibitor
    3. Decrease in monoamines or increase in β receptors

PARKINSON's DA AGONISTS	LEVODOPA [131]	CARBIDOPA [132]	BROMOCRIPTINE [133]	PERGOLIDE [134]	AMANTADINE [135]	DEPRENYL [136] (Selegiline)
	Oral Dopamine precursor Dopamine agonist	Blocks Conversion of L-DOPA to DA in periphery • Reduces side effects	DA agonist DA inhibits prolactin secretion	DA agonist Longer lasting	Release any DA left in nerve terminal	May arrest or retard progress of Parkinson's
	Crosses the BBB and is converted to DA by L-DOPA decarboxylase DA does NOT cross BBB	Inhibits Peripheral L-DOPA decarboxylase	**USE** • Hyperprolinemia		Block reuptake of DA from synapse	Works best with L-DOPA
	ON – OFF EFFECT Good for most days, then becomes IMMOBILE • Give Drug Holidays	**USE** Parkinson's Dis. L-DOPA + CARBIDOPA	**SIDE EFFECTS** • Nausea • Vomiting • Tachycardia • Erythromelalgia (red, painful, swollen feet)		**USE** • Antiviral agent but improves Parkinson's symptoms	MPTP $\rightarrow$ MPP $\rightarrow$ Parkinson's disease MAO-B
	WEARING OFF • After 5 – 8 yrs No longer effective Save as last treatment		• Mental change, schizophrenic			Must be given with L-DOPA
	SIDE EFFECTS 1. Emesis Vomiting, DA receptors 2. Tachycardia, arrhythmia 3. Orthostatic hypotension DA – splanchnic's 4. Hallucination, behavioral Δ, depression, confusion 5. Dyskinesia 6. Choreoathetosis face		**MECHANISM** Directly activates CNS DA receptors			Inhibits MAO-B metabolism MPTP inactive

ACETYLCHOLINE ANTAGONIST	ATROPINE [137]	BENZTROPINE [138]	TRIHEXYPHENIDYL [139] (THA)	DIPHENHYDRAMINE [140] (Benadryl®)
	Too many side effects for use here	**USE** • Drug-induced Parkinson's • Parkinson's if L-Dopa does not work **SIDE EFFECTS** • Sedation		

PARKINSON'S DISEASE

• ↓ DA
• ↑ ACh
Relative to each other

PHARMACOLOGIC CAUSES
1. DEMEROL®
• Synthetic heroin
• MPTP destroys DOPA nerves (dec DA)
2. ANTIPSYCHOTICS
• DOPA antagonist: HALOPERIDOL
                                CHLORPROMAZINE
(Block DA receptors)

HUNTINGTON'S CHOREA

• ↑ DA
• ↓ ACh
Relative to each other

HALOPERIDOL
• Treat Huntington's Chorea

ANTI-CONVULSANTS	PHENYTOIN	PHENOBARBITAL	CARBAMAZEPINE
	125	126	127
	First drug to show • Antiepileptic activity with NO sedation Inhibits spreading from focus of electrical discharge Prevents closing of Na channels Inhibits high frequency activity • NO block of initial discharge	MECH OF ACTION • Inc seizure threshold • Direct effect on membrane Major problem with sedation	Oral only USE • Trigeminal neuralgia • Tonic-clonic seizure
	LESS SEDATION	SIGNIFICANT SEDATION	LESS SEDATION
	INDICATED FOR • Tonic-clonic seizures (all seizures except 2:) • NOT with absence seizure • NOT with petit mal SIDE EFFECTS 1. Impairs cerebellar-vestibular integration • Nystagmus • Ataxia • Incoordination Blood Conc > 20 µg/ml May be irreversible 2. Dyskinesia • Reversible 3. Gum hyperplasia 4. Hypertrichosis 5. Coarse facial features (thickening of lips) 6. Teratogenic Fetal Phenytoin Syndrome • Cleft palate • Hair lip 7. Peripheral neuropathy 8. Megaloblastic anemia	Behavioral problems: •hyperactivity in children and elderly	NO cosmetic problems One of first choices SIDE EFFECTS • Nausea • Headache • Skin rash Start at low dose MAJOR PROBLEM • Aplastic anemia • Agranulocytosis • Water retention Safest – pregnancy

PREGNANCY

Both epilepsy and drugs used to treat it, cause fetal defects.
If on the drug and remove it
• Inc frequency of seizures

Use CARBAMAZEPINE and do NOT come off it

VALPROIC ACID – teratogenic

VALPROIC ACID [128]	ETHOSUXIMIDE [129]	TRIMETHADIONE[130]
Broad spectrum	Specific for Absence seizure	TX Absence seizures
USE • Absence seizure • Tonic-Clonic seizure Monotherapy		Too many side effects
	TOXICITY SIDE EFFECTS • Nausea	
Enhances GABA inhibition	• Sedation • Anorexia	
SIDE EFFECTS 1. Nausea 2. Inc body weight – satiety center 3. Hepatic failure – major problem in children 4. Acute pancreatitis 5. Teratogenic – neural tube defect – spina bifida	• Hiccupping • Headaches Inc frequency of grand mal seizures Tolerance for benzodiazepines	

SEIZURES

1. PARTIAL – local, restricted area
   a. Simple partial = without loss or impairment of consciousness, numb, tingle, locally reflected disturbance, seconds to minutes, Jacksonian variant.
   b. Complex partial = impairment of consciousness (most common in adults), stereotyped movements, confusion, Δ EEG of temporal lobe.

2. GENERALIZED – throughout the brain
   a. Nonconvulsive:
      Absence seizures = petit mal, stops and stares, Children < 8 yrs old, ends at about 15 yrs.
   b. Convulsive:
      Tonic-clonic = grand mal, scream, brief cry, tonic contractions, clonic, postictal depression, confusion, drowsiness.
      Status Epilepticus = tonic–clonic, continuous, repeated, life threatening.

TREATMENT

1. PARTIAL and GENERAL TONIC-CLONIC
   • CARBAMAZEPINE • PHENOBARBITAL • PRIMIDONE

2. ABSENCE SEIZURES
   • VALPROIC ACID • ETHOSUXIMIDE

3. STATUS EPILEPTICUS
   • BENZODIAZEPINE e.g. IV DIAZEPAM (Valium®)
   – short duration (D.O.C.), followed by PHENYTOIN

ANALEPTICS (CONVULSANTS)	DOXAPRAM [119]	NIKETHAMIDE [120]	PENTYLENETETRAZOL [121]	STRYCHNINE [122]	PICROTOXIN [123]	BICUCULLINE [124]
	USE Stimulate respiration in: 1. Postanesthetic respiratory depression 2. Chronic Obstructive Pulmonary Disease (COPD)		PTZ Reduces effects of GABA (-) • Causes CNS excitability	Poison Specific antagonist of Glycine (-) Blocks Glycine receptors	GABA antagonist Inhibits GABA at all levels	A research tool Competitive antagonist of GABA at the GABA receptor
		RARELY USED	USE DDx: epilepsy • Seizures	Profound convulsions	Presynaptic effect Closes Cl- channels where GABA receptors are linked	
			Potent convulsant	NO therapeutic value	(GABA works by inc influx of Cl- • Hyperpolarizes)	
				OD – Poisoning ℞ Strychnine Poisoning 1. DIAZEPAM 2. GLYCINE	BENZODIAZEPINES • Enhance GABA	
	ALL ENHANCE EXCITATION		ALL ARE CNS STIMULANTS			

ANTIANXIETY DRUGS NONBENZODIAZEPINES	PROPANEDIOL [154] CARBAMATES	ANTIHISTAMINE [155]	β BLOCKERS [156]	BUSPIRONE [157]	BARBITURATES [158]
	MEPROBAMATE TYBAMATE CRISOPRODOL	DIPHENHYDRAMINE (Benadryl®) HYDROXYZINE	PROPRANOLOL		PHENOBARBITAL
GENERAL • Excessive sedation • Significant drug interactions • Poor safety • Drug abuse	Does NOT act via GABA Effect is between BARB and BENZODIAZEPINES NOT USED CLINICALLY	Strong sedative Minor antianxiety HYDROXYZINE • Use for anxious addicts suffering from withdrawal	**USE** • Chronic anxiety • Debilitating anxiety • Stage fright Reduces autonomic NS symptoms associated with anxiety • Dec tremors • Dec sweating • Dec tachycardia Does NOT impair mental function	New Does NOT interact with other CNS depressants Acts on dopamine synapses Binds 5-HT receptors NO sedation NOT anticonvulsant NOT muscle relaxer Minimal abuse potential Mechanism unknown	NOT good NOT justified for antianxiety Opens Cl- channel longer (BDZ: Opens Cl- channels wider, more intensely) Induces microsomal enzymes • Dec effect with use over time • Inc tolerance Inhibits CNS CO_2 receptors • Respiratory depression Suppresses REM Suppresses Phase 4 Rebound insomnia Hypothermia SIDE EFFECT Porphyria

ANTIANXIETY DRUGS — LONG ACTING BENZODIAZEPINES

	CHLORDIAZEPOXIDE [143] (Librium®)	DIAZEPAM [144] (Valium®)	CHLORAZEPATE [145]	PRAZEPAM [146] (Centrax®)	FLURAZEPAM [147] (Dalmane®)
SEDATIVES	Oral $T_{1/2}$ = 2 – 4 days USE Alcohol withdrawal NOT used as sedative/hypnotic	Oral $T_{1/2}$ = 36 hr $T_{1/2}$ Long because of elimination • Rapid and extensive distribution in adipose tissue Active metabolites Very lipid soluble Short duration USE Status Epilepsy • Antianxiety • Sedative/Hypno • Muscle relaxant	$T_{1/2}$ = 2 days Some partial seizures		Oral $T_{1/2}$ = 60 hrs Duration = 7 – 10 days Many metabolites Very long lasting

> **General Structure**
> Phenol ring is substituted in the 5 position by halogen (electroneg group)

SHORT ACTING BENZODIAZEPINES

	ALPRAZOLAM [148] (Xanax®)	HALAZEPAM [149]	LORAZEPAM [150] (Ativan®)	OXAZEPAM [151]	TEMAZEPAM [152]	TRIAZOLAM [153]
SEDATIVES	$T_{1/2}$ = 12 – 15 hr	$T_{1/2}$ = 14 hr	$T_{1/2}$ = 16 hr Intermediate acting Safe to use with liver cirrhosis CONTRAINDICATED Narrow Angle Glaucoma	$T_{1/2}$ = 15 hr Safe to use with liver cirrhosis	$T_{1/2}$ = 10 hr Kidney excretion Overnight use	$T_{1/2}$ = 1.5 – 5 hr Peak = 1 – 2 hr ↓ Insomnia METABOLISM • 1st Pass Effect Hydroxylated and Conjugated • Hepatic microsomal oxidation Rebound insomnia

> **EARLY MORNING INSOMNIA**
> May be due to suspension because of rapid disappearance

> **REBOUND INSOMNIA**
> Abrupt discontinuation
> Short acting BDZ
> • Greater degree of tolerance develops

ANTIANXIETY DRUGS - GENERAL INFORMATION

MECHANISM OF ACTION
- Facilitates the inhibitory effect of GABA
- Allosteric Δ in GABA Rec complex
- Inc Cl⁻ conduction – hyperpolarizes
- GABA is required for BDZ function
- Compare with BARB, which just prolongs the opening of Cl⁻ channel
- BDZ intensifies the Cl⁻ flux channel

ANIMAL EXPERIMENTS
- Reduces the suppressive effects of punishment in animals
- Dec awareness
- Dec anxiety

CNS EFFECTS
1. ANXIOLYTIC • Impairs cortical input to reticular activating system
   - Suppress after discharge of limbic system
2. SEDATIVE / HYPNOTIC • More useful than BARBs • Dose response curve less steep
3. ANTICONVULSANT • Use: Status Epilepticus (D.O.C. –Valium®) • Inc seizure threshold
4. MUSCLE RELAXANT • IV

PERIPHERAL EFFECTS
- Safe
- Slight Dec in respiration
- Dec BP°, Dec LV stroke volume
- Slight tachycardia

OTHER USES (besides anxiety)
1. Alcohol withdrawal (Librium®)
2. Insomnia
3. Preanesthesia
4. Cardioversion
5. Tetanus
6. Neuromuscular disorders
7. Obstetrics – labor
8. Endoscopy
9. Prophylaxis of seizures

TOLERANCE
- Low level induction liver microsomal enzymes
- Short acting BDZs have a greater degree of tolerance
- Cross tolerance with other CNS Depress like BARB, Alcohol; Requires an increased dose

SLEEP
- All suppress Stage IV sleep
- Minor REM suppression without REM rebound

PHARMACOKINETICS
- Well absorbed orally
- Peak = 1 hr
- High lipid solubility
- High plasma protein bind > 85%
- Volume of distribution – Large
- Metabolized to active compounds – Inc the $T_{1/2}$
- Rapid redistribution in brain and fat tissue
- Oxidation and conjugation in liver is slow
- Excretion from kidney
- High therapeutic index

DRUG INTERACTION
1. CIMETIDINE
2. DISULFIRAM
3. ORAL CONTRACEPTIVES
4. ISONIAZID
   BDZ – Inhibits metabolism – Inc $T_{1/2}$

Heavy smoking – Dec BDZ effect

BDZ effects are additive with BARBs and Alcohol Inc CNS depression

WITHDRAWAL
- May not be seen for 5 – 7 days
- Longer $T_{1/2}$ – less withdrawal

SIDE EFFECTS
- Drowsiness
- Nausea
- Dec Libido
- Impaired cognition esp with elderly
- Paradoxical inc in anxiety
- Teratogenic
- Ataxia
- Rash at higher conc
- Confusion

WITH CHRONIC USE
- Tolerance to all effects and side effects except antianxiety action

ANTIPSYCHOTIC DRUGS (NEUROLEPTIC)	PHENOTHIAZINES [159]		
	CHLORPROMAZINE (Thorazine®)	THIORIDAZINE (Mellaril®)	TRIFLUOPERAZINE
DOPAMINERGIC ANTAGONISTS	Highly lipid soluble (Aliphatic) Low potency > 60 Breakdown prods > 90% Plasma bound < 60% Bioavailability Vol Dist > 7 L/kg (high) $T_{1/2} = 10 - 20$ hr 7 OH derivatives Inc autonomic side effects	A Piperazine High potency Dec autonomic side effects Fewer extrapyramidal side effects	
SYSTEMIC SIDE EFFECTS	EARLY: Rigidity, tremors, torticollis, grimacing, akathisia LATE: Stereotypical sucking movement, tardive dyskinesia		SIDE EFFECTS • Retinitis pigmentosa if dose > 800 mg/dl • Photosensitive rash
Oversedation	+++ (common)	+++ (common)	+ (rare)
Autonomic SE	+++ (common)	+++ (common)	+ (rare)
Extrapyramidal SE	++ (uncommon)	+ (rare)	+++ (common)
	High Dose Low Potency Inc Autonomic Effect Dec Neurologic Effect ←		⟵
	CHLORPROMAZINE • Anticholinergic ACh • Antihistamine • α adrenergic block (NE) • 5-HT blocker • DA blocker AUTONOMIC SIDE EFFECTS • Hypotension • Constipation • GI Ileus CPZ ALONE • No sleep or stupor CPZ + MORPH/BARB • Hypnotic DA RECEPTOR BLOCK • Antipsychotic DEC ACTIVITY • Sedate	NEUROLEPTICS CONTRAINDICATED Alcohol Withdrawal • Dec convulsion threshold • Mild anxiety state Acute brain syndrome	

	THIOXANTHENES [160]		BUTYROPHENONES [161]
FLUPHENAZINE	**THIOTHIXENE (Navane®)**		**HALOPERIDOL (Haldol®)**

Less sedation
Less autonomic
  blocking
More severe SE
  Extrapyramidal
	Low potency		Rapidly absorbed completely
			Peak level 2 – 5 hr
			Slowly excreted
			< 50% first week
			
			USE
			Emergency Tx of violent psychosis
			Few autonomic NS problems
			  (hypotension) (hypothermia)
			Weak antihistamine
			D.O.C. – heart disease

TOXICITY – Tardive dyskinesia			SIDE EFFECTS • Mastalgia • Lactation • Hyperpyrexia • Persistent tardive dyskinesia
+ (rare) + (rare) +++(common)	+++ (common) ++ (uncommon) ++ (uncommon)		–– + (rare) +++ (common)
		⟶	Low Dose High Potency Dec Autonomic Effect Inc Neurologic Effect

			High potency has an Inc
			  extrapyramidal side effect
			Minimal sedation
			TX
			  Huntington's Chorea
			  Tourette's Syndrome

ANTI PSYCHOTICS 2

RESERPINE [162]	LITHIUM CARBONATE [163]

RESERPINE [162]

Alkaloid from
  Rauwolfia serpentina
• Very potent
• Oral – absorbed well
  from the GI tract
• Antihypertensive
• Long lasting, Single
  dose has duration of
  action: several days

RESERPINE depletes
  NE and 5-HT, from
  natural stores

AUTONOMIC NS
Inc central parasymp
• Pupil constriction
  (miosis)
• Dec HR
• Inc GI activity
Dec central sympa-
  thetics (sympatholytic)
• Epigastric disease
• diarrhea
Antihypertensive

TOXICITY May lead to
  mental depression and
  suicidal tendencies
SIDE EFFECTS Sedation,
  drowsiness, lethargy
  (without sleep)

RESERPINE DEPRESSION
  can be countered by
  DOPA

CLOZARIL
  a new neuroleptic
• NO tardive
  dyskinesia character-
  istic of the other
  neuroleptics
• Causes: severe
  sedation, salivation,
  ortho hypotension
• Major side effect:
  agranulocytosis

LITHIUM CARBONATE [163]

Taken up rapidly – absorbed
Indicated in manic episodes of bipolar disorder
Dec mania

MANIA
1. Dec emotional ability   4. Pressured speech
2. Dec need for sleep   5. Overactivity
3. Flight of ideas   6. Involved in activities that can be
                               painful

EFFECTIVELY TREAT
• Elation, grandiosity, persecution, flight of ideas,
  expansiveness, irritability, manipulativeness, anxiousness
LESS EFFECTIVE
• Sleep problems, pressured speech, Inc motor activity,
  violence, distractible
MECHANISM
• Li^+ will displace Na^+ in transport system of CNS and kidney
• Interferes with transmitter properties of NE induced cAMP
  formation
• Dec excitability
TOXICITY
Anorexia, nausea, vomiting, thirst, loose stool (diarrhea), polyuria,
edema, goiter, fine tremor, twitches, weakness, unsteady gait,
slurred speech, drowsy, hyperreflexia, seizure, coma

VERY NARROW THERAPEUTIC INDEX

KINETICS
Acute dose: 1800 – 3600 mg/day,
Chronic dose: 600 – 1200 mg/day
mEq dose = 0.5 mg/kg/day, 300 mg = 8 mEq
Css = 0.5 – 1.2 mEq/L
Bioavailability = 100%, Plasma Protein Binding = 0
$T_{1/2}$ = 20 hr,
Vol Dist = 0.6 l/kg female, 0.7 l/kg male
Clearance = 20% Ccr
Li^+ plus NSAID (Ibuprofen)
• Alters blood flow in the kidney
• Causes an Inc conc Li^+ in blood
Caffeine effects: NO tea or coffee, Li^+ in depressed patient.
To relieve depression – drink coffee – swing from
hypomania ↔ depression

Most common cause of nephrogenic diabetes insipidus

CONTRAINDICATED
1. PREGNANCY – Cardiovasc abnormal baby
2. RENAL and CARDIAC disease
3. NONSTEROIDAL ANTI-INFLAM DRUGS
4. DIURETICS

Dec Seizure Threshold

MESCALINE (Amphetamines) [164]
• Similar structures to catecholamines • Causes paranoid schizophrenia

GENERAL INFORMATION ABOUT
ANTIPSYCHOTIC DRUGS

GENERAL ANTIPSYCHOTICS
1. Dec psychomotor agitation
2. Dec anxiety, hostility, fear
3. Dec aggressive, assaultive
4. Dec hallucinations
5. Dec confusion
6. Dec mania

Produce a feeling of
indifference toward the
environment, without
impairing sensorium and
without producing dysarthria
or ataxia

NEUROLEPTIC
ANIMALS:
1. Dec spontaneous movement
2. Dec complex behavior
3. NO effect on spinal reflex or
   unconditional escape response

HUMAN:
1. Dec initiative
2. Dec interest
3. Dec display of emotions
4. Dec range of affect
5. Dec conditioned avoidance (low dose)

SITE	DRUG EFFECT (to DA)
1. Limbic	Antipsychotic
2. Nigrostriatal	Parkinsonism
3. Tuberoinfundibular	Prolactin release, Hypothermia
4. CTZ	Antiemetic

ANTICHOLINERGIC
1. Loss of accommodation
2. Dry mouth
3. Difficulty in urination
4. Constipation – ileus
5. Tachycardia

ANTIADRENERGIC
1. Orthostatic hypotension
2. Impotent – Impaired ejaculation
3. Poikilothermy – ambient T°
4. Hyperthermia
5. ANS Effect > in low potency

TOXICITY
1. Sedation
2. Extrapyramidal effects
 • Parkinsonism
 • Acute torsion dystonia
 • Akathisia
 • Tardive dyskinesia
3. Autonomic blockade
 • Orthostatic hypotension
 • Dry mouth, tachycardia,
   Blurred vision, urinary
   retention, constipation
4. Neuroendocrine
 • Delayed ovulation, menses
 • Amenorrhea, galactorrhea,
 gynecomastia, edema, weight gain
 • Dec libido
5. Bone marrow depression
6. Ophthalmic pigmentation
7. Allergic effects: photosensitivity
8. Cholestatic jaundice

THERAPEUTIC USES
1. Schizophrenia 1° treatment
2. Acute psychosis
3. Amphetamine + LSD induced psychosis
4. Organic brain syndromes
5. Huntington's chorea
6. Intractable hiccups
7. Anesthetic adjunct, PostOp sedation
8. Antiemetic

SITES OF ACTION
1. Subcortical Retic formation
   (Inc filtering – dec stim)
2. Limbic system (DA site)
3. Basal ganglia (DA site)
4. Hypothalamus (DA site)

DOPAMINERGIC PATHWAYS
1. Mesolimbic – emotional
2. Nigrostriatal – movement
3. Tuberoinfundibular
   – secrete pituitary hormones

NEUROMUSCULAR JUNCTION BLOCKERS	
COMPETITIVE BLOCKERS (NON-DEPOLARIZING) [178]	**NON-COMPETITIVE BLOCKERS (DEPOLARIZING)** [179]

MECH reversibly compete with ACh for endplate nicotinic receptor, ganglionic blockade, histamine release
Dec threshold • Dec contraction • Paralysis
 	
Reversed by:
1. Cholinesterase inhibitors: Edrophonium & Neostigmine
2. Tetanic stimuli – enhances transmitter secretion
 	
SIX SPECIFIC AGENTS
1. d-TUBOCURARINE (CURARE)
  • Blocks neuromuscular junction
  • Ganglionic blockade
  • Releases histamine and heparin
    Bronchospasm, Dec BP°,
    Dec coagulation of blood
  • Hypotension and Δ HR
  • NOT metabolized
  • Slowly excreted in bile and urine
2. DIMETHYLTUBOCURARINE
  • 4 times more potent than Curare
  • Less ganglionic blocking and histamine release
  • NOT metabolized
3. GALLAMINE
  • about 1/5 as potent as Curare
  • Much less ganglionic blocking
  • Vagolytic, Stimulates sympathetic NS
    – Inc HR, Inc BP°
  • 100% kidney excretion
4. PANCURONIUM
  • Steroid, 6 times more potent than Curare
  • NO ganglionic block
  • Suppresses catecholamine uptake
  • NO histamine release
  • Metabolized and excreted in the urine
5. VERCURONIUM – analog of Pancuronium
  • Shortest acting competitive blocker
  • 6 times more potent than Curare
  • No ganglionic block
  • NO histamine release
  • Bile excretion
6. ATRACURIUM
  • Commonly used in U.S.
  • Breaks down in patients with kidney and liver failure
  • Based on pH and T° (Hoffman degradation) dec dose in heart surgery – cool body
  • One metabolite can cross the BBB – seizures
	MECHANISM
	  Combines with ACh receptors
	  Causes activation and current flow (enhanced by ACh)
	  Phase 1 – Depolarization block
	    • Fasciculations
	    • Inc intragastric P°
	    • Inc intraocular P°
	    • PostOp muscle pain
	  Phase 2 – Desensitization block (nonresponsive)
	
	SUCCINYLCHOLINE
	  • Widely used
	  • NOT selective for end plate receptors
	  • Will excite ganglia & neuroreceptors (arrhythmia)
	  • Inc plasma K⁺ conc
	  • Cardiac arrest
	  • Prolonged block
	  • Pseudocholinesterase deficit
	
	A treatment that increases ACh
	  • Enhances block
	Depolarizing noncompetitive blockers are antagonized by nondepolarizing competitive blockers

COMMON FEATURES OF
NEUROMUSCULAR JUNCTION BLOCKERS

- Poor lipid solubility
- Volume of distribution = blood volume
- Doesn't cross BBB or placental barriers
- Must be given IV
- Major action at nicotinic receptors, motor end plates
- Also at ACh receptors, CNS, and muscarinic receptors
- Paralysis first detected in face muscles,
- Respiratory muscle affected last
- Never give in absence of artificial respiration
- Pharm action terminated by diffusion from site of action
    (except Succinylcholine)

IDEAL GENERAL ANESTHESIA

1. Analgesia
2. Dec consciousness
3. Skeletal muscles relax
4. Loss of undesirable reflexes
5. Amnesia

MAJOR USES OF NEUROMOTOR JUNCTION BLOCKERS

- Adjunct to general anesthesia
- Dec mech resistance of chest wall for artificial respirator
- Symptomatic treatment of convulsive states
- Alignment of fractures

INTERACTIONS
1. Inhaled anesthetics augment block

ISOFLURANE HALOTHANE N_2O, OPIOIDS
ENFLURANE   BARBITURATES

2. Antibiotics
3. Local anesthetics and antiarrhythmics
4. Depolarizing blockers are antagonized by non-depolarizing blockers

HISTAMINE [165]	CLASSIC ANTIHISTAMINES [166]

• Synthesized from histidine in many tissues
• Stored in granules, mast cells, and basophil cells
• Release triggered – many stimuli
• Non-mast cell histamine – CNS Hypothalamus – T° regulation
 	
RECEPTORS
1. Bronchiolar smooth muscle H_1
  • bronchoconstriction (asthma)
2. GI smooth muscle H_1
  • contraction (diarrhea)
3. Other smooth muscle
  • uterine contraction (abortion)
4. Nervous system H_1
  • nerve ending (pain, itching)
5. Cardiovascular H_1, H_2
  • vasodilate (Dec BP°, Inc HR)
  • Inc permeability (edema)
6. Triple response H_1, H_2
  • redness, wheal, flare
7. GI Secretion H_2
  • parietal cell – gastric acid
 	
Histamine • No therapeutic use
 	
BETAZOLE
• Isomer of histamine
• Formerly used to Tx gastric acid secretion (atrophic gastritis)
 	
PENTAGASTRIN
• Now used
• More selective for H_2 receptors
	1. Ethanolamines
	  • DIPHENHYDRAMINE (Itch)
	  • DIMENHYDRINATE
	2. Ethylenediamine
	  • TRIPELENNAMINE
	3. Alkylamine
	  • CHLORPHENIRAMINE
	4. Piperazine derivatives
	  • MECLIZINE • CYCLIZINE
	5. Phenothiazine derivative
	  • PROMETHAZINE

	Highly lipid soluble
	Orally – well absorbed
	Distributed widely (even CNS)
	All penetrate the CNS blood-brain-barrier
	
	BLOCKS RECEPTORS
	 H_1, H_2, α, muscarinic, 5-HT, and local anesthetic
	ANTI-H_1 EFFECTS
	1. Dec vasodilation
	2. Treat asthma – Dec bronchoconstriction
	  (NOT effective with allergic asthma)
	3. Antidiarrheal – mostly parasymp,
	  Dec smooth muscle contraction
	(above 3 properties are NOT USED)
	4. Stop pain and itch
	  DIPHENHYDRAMINE Ointment
	ANTIMUSCARINIC RECEPTOR EFFECTS
	 (like SCOPOLAMINE)
	1. Sedation
	2. Anti-motion sickness caused by vestibular disturbances
	LOCAL ANESTHETIC
	 • DIPHENHYDRAMINE • PROMETHAZINE
	α ADRENERGIC BLOCK
	 • Orthostatic hypotension
	ANTIEMETIC PROMETHAZINE
	 • Nausea, vomiting associated with pregnancy
	 • May be TERATOGENIC
	NOT EFFECTIVE against common cold virus
	SIDE EFFECTS (vary with purpose)
	1. If use for pain & itching, SE: sedation
	2. If use for sleep aid, SE: dry mouth, blurred vision
	ACUTE POISONING CNS excitement
	OD: CNS stimulation
	1. Hallucination 4. Convulsions
	2. Excitation 5. Death
	3. Ataxia

NEW ANTI HISTAMINES [166]	
H$_1$ ANTIHISTAMINES [167]	**H$_2$ ANTIHISTAMINES** [169]
TERFENADINE ASTEMIZOLE	CIMETIDINE (CTD) RANITIDINE (RTD) FAMOTIDINE (FTD) NIZATIDINE (NTD)
Can't penetrate BBB Fewer side effects USES 1. Urticaria 2. Atopic dermatitis 3. Allergic rhinitis 4. Stop pain and itching NOT EFFECTIVE IN TREATING • Cold (Virus) • Allergic asthma SIDE EFFECT • Sedation • Dry mouth	Blocks GI secretion, Dec gastric acid and pepsin INDICATIONS 1. ULCERS: peptic, gastric, duodenal 2. Zollinger-Ellison syndrome • High dose 3. URTICARIA (speculative) When DIPHENHYDRAMINE is ineffective CIMETIDINE • Older of the new drugs • Less potent MORE SIDE EFFECTS 1. ANTIANDROGENIC • Gynecomastia • Galactorrhea • Decreased libido 2. Leukocytopenia (Dec WBC) 3. Confusion 4. Lethargy 5. Inhibits cytochrome P$_{450}$ enzymes RANITIDINE (RTD) FAMOTIDINE (FTD) NIZATIDINE (NTD) • Fewer side effects • NO antiadrenergic effects • NO antiandrogen effects • Long term, large dose inhibits Cyt P$_{450}$ enzymes RTD • Much less P$_{450}$ effect, leukocytopenia, too FTD and NTD not reported FTD • Most potent

CROMOLYN [168]

Prevents histamine release from storage granules of basophil and mast cells

---

ANTIHISTAMINE USES

1. STOP PAIN AND ITCHING
   Atopic dermatitis
   DIPHENHYDRAMINE
2. CHRONIC URTICARIA – *NEW*
3. ALLERGIC RHINITIS – *NEW*
4. SEDATIVE – *CLASSIC*
5. MOTION SICKNESS – *CLASSIC*
6. NAUSEA, VOMITING – *CLASSIC*

ANTIHISTAMINE PROPERTIES
(CLASSIC AND NEW)

1. ANTI H$_1$ • Dec vasodilation • NO Dec BP°
   • Dec bronchoconstriction • Dec smooth
   muscle contraction • Dec pain and itching
   (CLASSIC ONLY)
2. ANTIMUSCARINIC
   CNS • Dec nausea, vomit, motion sickness
     • Dec Parkinson's • Sedation
   PNS • Anticholinergic
3. LIPID SOLUBILITY
     • Crosses BBB (CNS) • sedation
   (New drugs can NOT cross BBB)
4. α BLOCK • Orthostatic hypotension
5. LOCAL ANESTHETIC RECEPTOR ACTION

ANTIEMETICS (4 CLASSES)[173]	ANTIDOPAMINERGICS[174]

First ID cause before Tx
  (i.e. intestinal obstruction needs surgery,
    not drugs)
PROBLEMS
• Dehydration
• Electrolyte imbalance
• Esophageal rupture
• Nutritional deficiency
• Can't take oral medication
	CHLORPROMAZINE (Thorazine®)
	PROCHLORPERAZINE (Compazine®)
	HALOPERIDOL (Haldol®)

INDICATIONS Vomiting due to: 1. Anesthesia 2. Cancer chemotherapy 3. Radiation sickness 4. Motion sickness	Blocks dopaminergic receptors of chemoreceptor trigger zone **INDICATIONS** Nausea due to • Anesthesia • Chemotherapy • Radiation
ALL Other Types — Treat the cause or the emesis	NOT Effective • Vertigo • Motion Sickness
CONTRAINDICATION 1. Abdominal pathology • Intestinal block (treat surgically) 2. Inc intracranial pressure 3. Orthostatic hypotension 4. Migraine headaches	**SIDE EFFECTS** 1. Drowsiness – sedation 2. Orthostatic hypotension 3. Extrapyramidal effects • Dystonia • Akathisia • Parkinsonism 4. Blood dyscrasia

CAUSES OF EMESIS
1. Poisoning
2. Disease
  • GI
  • Meningeal
  • Migraine headaches
3. Drugs
  • Anticancer
  • Heroin OD
  • Emetics
4. Physical Stimuli
  • Motion sickness
  • Vertigo
  • Gag reflex
5. Psychological
  • Visual stimuli
  • Olfactory stimuli
6. Emotional upset
7. Endocrine
8. Visceral / Abdominal pain
	ANTIDOPAMINERGICS
	• Antipsychotic – high doses
	• Antiemetic – low doses
	
	Except THORAZINE
	• an antipsychotic, NOT an antiemetic

ANTIHISTAMINES [175]	ANTICHOLINERGICS [176]	MISCELLANEOUS [177]

DIPHENHYDRAMINE
  (Benadryl®)
• D.O.C.
• O.T.C. Hypnotic –
  very drowsy
DIMENHYDRINATE
  (Dramamine®)
PIPERAZINE (Cyclizine)
• Teratogenic
MECLIZINE (Marezine®)
PROMETHAZINE
  (Phenergan®)
 	
Blocks H_1 receptors in the
  vomiting center,
  histamine antagonist
 	
• NOT antipsychotic
• Less sedating
 	
Anticholinergic effect:
Antimuscarinic
• May also account for
  some antiemetic
 	
Also acts at chemoreceptor
  trigger zone
 	
1° USE Motion sickness
 	
SIDE EFFECTS
  (Anticholinergic SE)
1. Sedation – drowsiness
2. Blurred vision
3. Dry mouth
4. Urine retention
5. Constipation
 	
Antiemetic effect from:
1. Antimuscarinic
2. H_1 Antagonist
 	
PROMETHAZINE
  Tx: Anesthetic vomiting
	SCOPOLAMINE
	ATROPINE
	
	Nonselective muscarinic
	  receptor blockers
	
	MECHANISM
	1. Blocks cholinergic input
	   from the vestibular
	   apparatus to the
	   vomiting center
	2. Blocks CTZ
	3. Antispasmodic
	  • Dec GI motility
	
	USE
	Indicated for:
	  motion sickness
	
	SIDE EFFECTS
	1. Tachycardia
	2. Blurred vision
	3. Dry mouth
	4. Mydriasis
	5. Urinary retention
	
	SCOPOLAMINE – D.O.C.
	• Rapid onset
	• Short acting
	• Oral, SQ, or Patch
		DIPHENIDOL
		Acts at vestibular
		  apparatus and CTZ
		
		Effective for ALL types of
		  emesis
		No advantage in use
		
		SIDE EFFECTS
		1. Hallucinations, Auditory &
		   Visual
		2. Sedation / Drowsiness
		3. Parkinsonism
		4. Confusion
		
		TRIMETHOBENZAMIDE
		  Block DA receptors CTZ
		Δ^9 TETRAHYDRO-
		   CANNABINOL (Δ^9 THC)
		MARIJUANA
		Blocks opioid receptors in
		  forebrain and VC
		
		INDICATED emesis:
		1. Cancer chemotherapy
		2. If others don't work
		
		SIDE EFFECTS
		1. Sedation
		2. Dry mouth
		3. Dizziness
		4. Inability to concentrate
		
		NABILONE (Cesamet®)
		DRONABINOL
		
		METOCLOPRAMIDE
		  (Reglan®)
		Blocks DA receptors CTZ
		• Peripheral stimulant,
		   ACh release
		• Sensitizes GI smooth muscle
		• Restores GI motility
		• Inc contraction sm muscle
		• Prevents esophagus reflux
		
		SIDE EFFECTS
		1. Sedation 2. Fatigue
		3. Headache
		
		NOT EFFECTIVE
		• Motion sickness
		• Labyrinthine disorders

EMETICS [170]	IPECAC [171]	APOMORPHINE [172]
EMESIS Function: protective Vomiting is a symptom of a disease, poison, drug side effect **SEQUENCE OF EVENTS** 1. PRELIMINARY EVENT – fast breathing, excessive salivation, mydriasis (pupils dilate), sweat, pallor, arrhythmia 2. RETCHING – deep inspiration, strong abdominal musc contract, contents in the esophagus (can go back down) 3. EMESIS (EXPURGATE) – rapid rise in intrathoracic P°, Inc contraction of abdominal muscle, expulsion **CAUSES** Physical, chemical, psychological **TYPES OF CAUSES** 1. PERIPHERAL – gag reflex, GI inflammation, visceral pain 2. CHEMICAL – drugs (morphine, anti-cancer drugs) – endocrine malfunction 3. VESTIBULAR – motion sickness, vertigo 4. MENINGEAL – rise in intracranial pressure 5. PSYCHOLOGICAL – cortical, visual, olfactory 6. LIMBIC – Emotional **INTEGRATION** VOMITING CENTER (VC) – medulla, dorsolateral reticular formation, near the 4th ventricle CHEMORECEPTOR TRIGGER ZONE (CTZ) – Area Postrema, sensory area that responds to drug outside BBB, high quantity of DA neurons	D.O.C. – Best, safe, oral (PO) EMETINE – active ingredient **MECH OF ACTION** • Stimulates CTZ • Gastric afferents (irritates stomach) Vomit in 30 min • More effective with water, Give 200 – 300 ml H_2O, Inc volume – Inc contract force of stomach (preload) **DOSE** Adult, 20 – 30 ml Child, 15 ml **SIDE EFFECT** Cardiotoxic in high quantity **CONTRAINDICATED** Child under 1 yr old	NOT as safe Very little analgesic effect **MECH OF ACTION** •DA agonist CTZ • Vomiting SQ: 0.12 mg/kg Adult 0.06 mg/kg Child More effective with water **SIDE EFFECTS** 1. Restlessness 2. Tremors 3. CNS depression gives rise to 4. 4. Respiratory depression If OD • Severe vomiting, Treat with NALOXONE

CONTRAINDICATIONS OF EMESIS
1. Shock, unconsciousness
2. Ingestion of caustic agent (Lye, Acid)
3. Petroleum poisoning
4. STRYCHNINE poisoning

ALTERNATIVES TO EMESIS
1. Gastric lavage
2. Activated charcoal

PROPERTIES OF LOCAL ANESTHETICS [194]

CLINICAL USES
1. Topical
2. Infiltrative
   a. Inject into tissue
   b. Spinal (subarachnoid)
   • Nerve roots
   • CNS toxicity
   c. Epidural – spinal nerves
   d. Brachial plexus
   e. IV • itching
   f. IV regional
   • retrograde exsanguinate

NERVES
C, Aδ · Pain (affected 1st)
B · Preganglionic
Aα · Fast myelinated
Aβ · Fast Aδ · pain
Aγ · Thin myelinated
C · Nonmyelinated
Low conc – mostly
sensory loss C, Aδ fibers

ORDER OF SENSITIVITY
1. Autonomic NS (C fibers)
   • Flushing, hyperemia,
     vasodilation
2. Temperature
   (Aδ and C fibers)
3. Pain (Aδ and C)
4. Touch / P° (Aα and Aβ)
5. Proprioception
   (Aα and Aβ)
6. Skeletal muscle activity

ANATOMIC SITE OF ACTION
1. Free nerve endings
2. Special sense receptor
   organs
3. Nonmyelinated fibers(C)
4. Node of Ranvier
5. Internodal segments

TWO WAYS TO DECREASE EXCITABILITY
1. DEPOLARIZE THE NERVE
2. MEMBRANE STABILIZATION – LOCAL ANESTHETIC
LOCAL ANESTHETICS
1. Membrane stabilization
   (not depolarization)
2. Remove Na+ current (Not K+)
3. NO specific receptors for
   LA – diffuse

ACTIVE FORM OF LA
LA are weak bases at pH 6.7
 – 99% ionized
   (PROCAINE, LIDOCAINE)
1% is nonionized, Nonionized
   form gets into axoplasm and
   ionizes, ION TRAPPING
Active Form: Both forms
Primarily the ionized form is
   the active form (for most)

MEMBRANE SITE OF ACTION
1. Outer surface (TETRACAINE)
2. Inner surface
3. In between surface
   membranes
   (PROCAINE, LIDOCAINE)
Ionized form – aqueous pores
Nonionized – dissolves into
   the lipid membrane
   • Permeable
   • Membrane expander

THEORIES OF ACTION
1. LA Competitive, Inhibits Na+,
   Na+ antagonist
2. LA Competitive, Inhibits Ca++
3. Anesthetic expands
   membrane
4. LA plugs into the Na+ channel

LA EFFECTS ON
PERIPHERAL NERVES
1. Dec Na+ current
2. Dec excitability
3. Dec action potential size
4. Decremental conduction
   3 – 4 nodes
5. Inc refractory period (40 x)
   • Nerve
   • Heart (antiarrhythmic)
6. Use dependent block
   (high frequency failure)
7. Conduction block

FACTORS WHICH
AFFECT INTENSITY
1. Concentration
2. Potency
3. pH of environment
   • Inflammation will lower
     pH, More difficult to
     diffuse · Ionized

DURATION
1. Inc concentration
   • Inc duration
2. Length of nerve exposed
3. Diffusibility of drug
   molecule
4. Vascularity of area
5. Volume of drug
   administered
6. Binding affinity (Inc)
   • Inc duration
7. Given with
   vasoconstrictor (EPI)
8. Intrinsic duration of drug
   itself
9. No or little metab at site

TOXICITY
1. Cardiovasc effects
   ECG: • Inc PR interval
        • Inc QRS duration
   Effects: • Dec CO, Dec BP°
        • Hypotension
        • Sympathetic paralysis
        • Arrhythmia
   Severe effects: • AV block
        • Asystole Sinus tachycardia
2. CNS effects:
        • Light-headedness
        • Dizziness • Tinnitus
        • Drowsiness
        • Disorientation
        • Depression
   Severe: Convulsions, Resp
   arrest, Seizures, Unconsciousness, Muscle twitch,
   Tremors, Skeletal muscle
   paralysis with high doses
3. Allergies • Esters
4. MeHb • Amides

$$\frac{\text{BUPIVACAINE}}{\text{TETRACAINE}} > \frac{\text{LIDOCAINE}}{\text{MEPIVACAINE}} > \text{PROCAINE}$$

LOCAL ANESTHETICS (ESTERS)	COCAINE [195]	PROCAINE (Novocain®) [196]	BENZOCAINE [197]	TETRACAINE [198]

Metabolized in the blood
 	
ADMINISTERED
Infiltrative (SQ)
Subdural
Epidural
	First clinically significant LA
	Plant • Chew leaves
	• Numbs mouth
	• CNS stimulant
	• Allays fatigue
	• Anorexia
	
	1800 – Crystallize LA
	1884 – Freud, Koller
	  – Eye surgery
	
	Should never be injected
	Topical Use Only
	4 – 10% conc
	• Seizures
	• Vasoconstriction
	• Rhinology
	• Corneal anesthetic
	• Before intubation
	• Prevents mucous
	  membrane bleeding
	• (+) Inotropic
	• (+) Chronotropic
	
	SIDE EFFECTS
	• Hypertension
	• Tachycardia
	• Arrhythmia
	• Psychic stimulus
		First successful LA
		Potency = 1
		Nerve Block (1 – 2%)
		Spinal anesthetic (5 – 20%)
		1000 mg maximum dose
		
		ADMIN Parenterally
		
		Duration = 1 hr
		Metabolic product is PABA
		which inhibits sulfonamides
		
		NOT for topical use
		Poor diffusion
		Nonionized / ionized
		channel blocker
		
		SIDE EFFECT Allergy
			TOPICAL Use Only
			
			No N in side chain
			• Low solubility
			• Does not penetrate
			  tissue
			No IV administration
			TOPICAL/ ORAL
			  – for burns
			
			Membrane expansion
			theory
			– Distortion of
			  membranes alters Na^+
			  channel function
			  Dec Na^+ flux
			  Nonionized
			  Only one active with no
			  charge
				Very powerful
				Long acting 4 – 10 hr
				BUTYL GROUP
				• Inc lipid solubility
				• Inc potency
				Dose 0.1 – 0.5 conc
				
				SIDE EFFECTS
				• Very quickly
				  Syncope / Toxicity
				  (NO Prodromal)
				• Spinal anesthesia
				  0.15 % solution
				  Max dose = 100 mg
				
				Most potent ester
				Longest lasting
				
				CNS
				• Coma and convulsion
				• Outer membrane
				  Na^+ blocker

ESTERS METABOLIZED
• in the Liver
• in the Plasma

Use Esters if have liver damage

LOCAL ANESTHETICS (AMIDES)	LIDOCAINE[199]	BUPIVACAINE[200]	MEPIVACAINE[201]	DIBUCAINE[202]	PRILOCAINE[203]
Metabolized in the Liver	Best overall local antiarrhythmic (IV) 1% Solution Max Dose = 300 mg Duration: 1 – 3 hr **USE** • Topically • Infiltrative • Spinal • Epidural Metabolized to over 100 compounds 2 may be convulsant, but LIDOCAINE is an anticonvulsant EPI + LIDOCAINE will increase duration from 1 to 4 hrs Nonionized / Ionized	Longest acting Duration 4 – 6 hr 0.05% conc – Higher doses can be given with vasoconstrictor Max Dose = 200 mg **SIDE EFFECTS** Cardiovascular • Toxicity Epidural • Arrhythmia **CONTRAINDICATED** Pregnancy	Very weak local Anesthetic Dental surgery • Heart patient • Do NOT need EPI Longer duration due to its own vasoconstrictor properties Max dose = 400 mg	Potent Max dose = 75 mg **USE** Hemorrhoids	**SIDE EFFECTS** • Methemoglobinemia • Hypoxia

GENERAL ANESTHETICS (INHALATION)	NITROUS OXIDE [180]	DIETHYL ETHER [181]	HALOTHANE [182]	ENFLURANE [183]	ISOFLURANE [184]	METHOXYFLURANE [185]
MAC (%)	101.0%	1.9%	1.4%	1.7%	0.8%	0.2%
Oil/Gas	(least soluble) 1.4	65.0	99	99	224	970 (most soluble)
Heart Rate	NO Δ	NO Δ	DEC	DEC	DEC	GASES Characteristics: 1. Bronchodilators 2. Dec Min Vent 3. Dec cerebrovascular resistance • Inc blood flow • Inc BP° head 4. (-) Inotropic Dec CO Dec contraction 5. Hyperthermia Large Inc T° Damages tissue Rigor – Heat Tx: Dantrolene 6. GABA and NIC ACh
Arrhythmia	NO	NO	YES – INC	INC (less severe)	YES – INC	
Catechol Sensitivity (cause arrhythmia)	NO Δ	NO Δ	YES – INC	YES	YES	
Cardiac Output	DEC	DEC	DEC	DEC	DEC	
Blood Pressure	NO Δ	DEC	DEC	NO Δ	DEC	
Liver Toxicity	NONE	NONE	YES – Br, Rare/Fatal	NONE	NONE	
Skeletal Muscle (synaptic transmission)	NO Δ	NO Δ	CURARE-like, mild	CURARE-like	CURARE-like	
Smooth Muscle	NO Δ	RELAX	RELAX Hypotension, Pheo	NO Δ	RELAX	
Analgesia	POTENT (fast) POOR (low lipid sol)	GOOD	NOT POTENT (slow), in blood (longer, more soluble)			EXTREMELY POTENT
Action/Duration	FAST (low blood sol)	SLOW			FASTER	
Explosive/Flame	NO (stable)	YES	NO			

GENERAL ANESTHETICS (INHALATION)	NITROUS OXIDE	DIETHYL ETHER	HALOTHANE	ENFLURANE	ISOFLURANE	METHOXYFLURANE
ADVANTAGES	Post Anesthetic Nausea, vomit rare N_2O + HALOTHANE N_2O – fast, short act HAL – longer acting, dissolves in blood	Stage IV (OD) – causes Resp arrest before CV arrest GOOD – can blow off excess ETHER	Hypotensive drug – Surgery PHEO Inhibits coughing and laryngospasm Dec bronchospasm Good for ASTHMA	More stable NO Br Less hypotensive Dec CO & HR BP° same – No effect on smooth muscle	Very stable NO preservative NO Br substitute Rapid induction Rapid recovery	Obstetrics
	Inc lipid solubility • Dec % MAC • Inc potency Δ MAC: Dec body T°, hypoxia, hypovol, Resp, or CO changes (MAC = 1 / Potency)		Vagomimetic – Dec HR (can cause arrhythmia)		Least metabolized NO breakdown NO liver toxicity	
DISADVANTAGES	Diffusion hypoxia (Give O_2 to remove) Inc P° – Low compli (Ear) Inc Vol – high compl (pneumothorax) TERATOGENIC	Common: Post anesthesia nausea and vomit Flammable, Explode Slow induction Slow recovery Vagolytic – but NO arrhythmia	Spontaneous Decomp Bromide release – Tissue toxicity Hepatotoxicity (rare, but fatal) $T_{1/2}$ = 1 week Allergy to preservative, Analog of Diethyl Ether + Chloroform	Causes EEG sign of convulsion Arrhythmia Nausea, vomiting in females **CONTRAINDICATED** Epileptics	Inc resp depression Pungent odor	Very high lipid solubility Difficult to control Nephrotoxic Most extensively metabolized Halogenated hydrocarbon

CONTRAINDICATED
• Pregnant • Allergic
Cause: Abortion, Nerve damage
(fetal) Malig hyperthermia

	CYCLOPROPANE	CHLOROFORM [186]
	Explosive Resp depression Post anesthesia nausea, vomiting (NOT USED)	Halogenated hydrocarbon Very hepatotoxic Anesthesia Stable

FOUR STAGES OF ANESTHESIA
I. Analgesia • Spinal cord, sensory loss
II. Delirium • Small inhibitory (GABA) neurons gone first
• Facilitates excitatory • Arrhythmia, seizures
(GO in and out of this stage as QUICKLY as possible)
III. Anesthesia •Retic activ sys and spinal reflex, Dec resp rate
IV. O.D. • Medullary resp and vasomotor centers • Critical

GENERAL ANESTHETICS (INTRAVENOUS)	THIOPENTAL[187]	OPIOIDS [188]	INNOVAR®[189]
	Sulfur derivative of barbituric acid 2.5% solution at pH 11 Soluble in alkaline media • precipitates if given too rapidly	MORPHINE	DROPERIDOL + FENTANYL • Neuroleptic sedative • Used with NO_2 to speed up
ADVANTAGES	Potent anesthesia Dec cerebral blood flow NO Inc intracranial pressure	Cardiac surgery	Neuroleptoanalgesia • Disinterest in the environment without loss of consciousness Anesthesia, but responsive • Conscious • Cooperate Antiemetic Speed induction with NO_2
DISADVANTAGES	Weak analgesic (Antianalgesic at low doses) Need local anesthetic with it Respiratory system • Irritant • Depressant Dec Laryngospasm Hypothermia Peripheral vasoconstrictor Muscle pain if given with depolarizing neuronal blocker (Succinylchol) CONTRAINDICATED Intermittent porphyria	Poor amnesia Severe PostOp respiratory depression	Antiadrenergic CONTRAINDICATED • Asthmatics • Myasthenia

KETAMINE [190]	ETOMIDATE [191]	BENZODIAZEPINE [192]	PROPANIDID [193]
Dissociative anesthetic "Angel Dust" Brief catatonia		DIAZEPAM LORAZEPAM Preanesthesia – Slow onset	Rapid acting (as THIOPENTAL) Metabolized by plasma cholinesterase
Amnesia Profound algesia, Antiarrhythmia Inc CO CNS stim of sympathetics USE Emergency Tx of shock patient • Do NOT need ventilator	Minimal cardiovasc or resp changes	Prolongs anesthesia Facilitates amnesia	Dec BP° Dec cardiac output
Emergence phenomenon • Bad "Trips" illusions • Pretreat with DIAZEPAM Inc intracranial pressure CONTRAINDICATED • HT patient • Stroke • CBL emboli	CAUSES Myoclonia without EEG Δ		Severe hypotension Induces seizures

IV AGENTS
1. Rapid induction
2. Recovery = redistribution away from site
3. Respiratory irritant
4. Highly lipid soluble
5. Must give IV slowly
6. Specific receptor action

PAIN

PAIN is felt when there is a stimulus great enough to cause tissue damage

- Mechanical – Break skin
- Chemical – Burn
- Thermal – (45°C)

RESPONSE TO PAIN

1. AUTONOMIC: (varies)
- Inc BP°
- Perspire, sweat
- Pale
- Diarrheal movement or constipation

2. SOMATIC
- Reflex removal (simple)
- Rub area (complex)

3. EMOTIONAL
- Anger, aversion, remembrance, frustration

MORPHINE: pain present, but does NOT afflict mind – Changes response

NONPHARMACOLOGIC MANAGEMENT

1. T.E.N.S.
2. Dorsal column stimulation
3. Implant electrodes in brain
4. Destructive lesion
5. Hypnosis
6. Acupuncture

PHARMACOLOGIC (ANALGESICS) MANAGEMENT

General Info
Pain is indefinable

Characteristics
- Where:
  Somatic vs Visceral
- Quality
- Intensity

Scale (analogy)
0 NO Pain
1 Mild
2 Moderate
3 Severe

Drug Selection
Depends on: Pain, Age,
Other Rx, Ulcer,
or where drug works

PAIN THRESHOLD – First feel pain

PAIN TOLERANCE – Can't stand pain

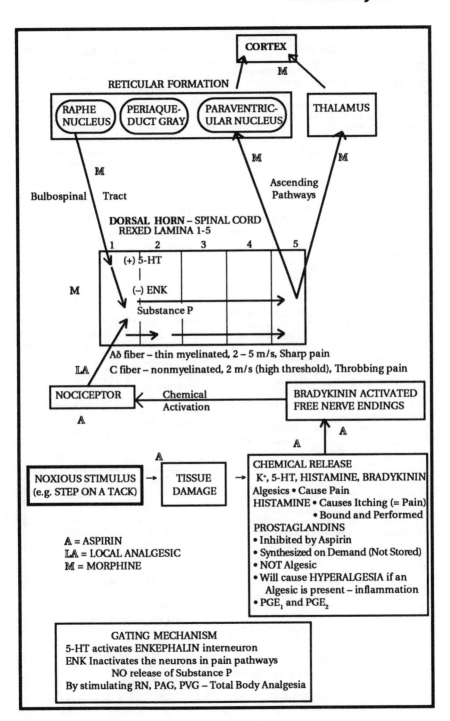

CENTRAL ANALGESICS

MORPHINE [204]	CODEINE [205]	MEPERIDINE (Demerol®) [206]
• From Far East Poppy plant (alkaloid) • Me group on N essential for activity • Without Me – inactive Normorphine • 5 Rings, phenolic OH, alcohol OH • Heroin – replace OHs with acetate (diacetyl morphine) • NOT more potent, just enters brain more quickly	• Natural ¹⁄₁₀ Potency • Me of phenolic OH • Duration = 4 hr • 60 mg starting dose	Oral absorption good Dose 300 mg, 2–3 hr • Relaxes smooth muscle • NO Miosis (constriction) • NO Histamine release • Active metabolite can cause grand mal seizures on inc dose • NOT antitussive • Prevent biliary colic, but NOT relieve it • Dec OPIOID craving

EFFECTS

1. Sedation
2. 80% euphoria (20% dysphoria)
3. Analgesia • Combines with central & peripheral opiate receptors
   • Reticular formation (important)
4. Myosis • stim Edinger-Westphal nucleus
5. Respiratory depression
   • 1° cause of death
   • Direct effect on medulla oblongata
   • Dec rate and depth of breathing
   • CO_2 is stimulus for breathing, Morphine directly blocks CO_2 activation
   • Peripheral drive remains intact, carotid body
     – Slower rate (If give pure O_2, stops breathing)
   • Inc P° CO_2 – Causes brain vessels to dilate
     – Inc CSF pressure
     (Contraindicated: brain damaged)
6. Antitussive • Dec cough center
7. Emetic Center • Vomit center
   • Direct effect VC – Antiemetic
   • Indirect effect CTZ – Emesis
8. Smooth muscle
   a. Bronchoconstriction • Cholinergic
     • Histamine release
   b. Gut • block peristalsis
     • Antidiarrheal / constipation
9. Urinary retention and urgency
10. Gall bladder
    • Constricts GB, Sphincter of Oddi, and Bile duct before pain relief occurs
    To Help: give Meperidine or Ca^{++} blockers
11. Releases histamine • bronchoconstrictor
    • curare-like effect
12. Formication • itching
13. Sweating

KINETICS

• 10 mg Oral dose • Not much effect
• Give IV, IM, SQ • Dec bioavailability
• Duration:
  3 – 4 hr, DON'T wait for pain to return
MORPHINE • Dec emotional response, feel pain, but do not care
• Inhibits Substance P
• Inc pain threshold • Inc pain tolerance
• Change input into nociceptors
  (In the spinal cord – dorsal horn)

EFFECTS (CODEINE)

• Antitussive
• Analgesia: acute pain
• Less addicting
• Constipation give MOM

CODEINE + AMPHETAMINE will increase analgesia

METHADONE [207]	PROPOXYPHENE [208]
• Good analgesic • Dose 15 mg • Long lasting, 15 hr • Substitute for OPIOID addiction 1 dose/day: • blocks craving • blocks euphoria	• Poor analgesic • Addictive d-PROPOX – analgesia (Darvon®) 1-PROPOX – antitussive (Navrod®)

DRUG DEPENDENCE

(MORPHINE-type dependence)
1. Overpowering desire for more
2. Inc tolerance to dose, except:
   a. Eye – Miosis (constriction)
   b. Gut – Inc constipation
   c. Histamine release – ↑ formation
3. Psychological Dependence
4. Physical Dependence
   Abstinence Syndrome
   – NO Seizures, NO Hallucination, NO Tolerance to miosis or constipation

TOLERANCE

• NOT due to kinetics
• DUE to receptors
• Takes 2 weeks

ENKEPHALIN [209] ENDORPHINS	PENTAZOCINE (Talwin®) [210]	DIPHENOXYLATE [211]	FENTANYL [212] (Sublimaze®)

PRO-OPIOCORTIN:
 • β ENDORPHIN
 • γ MSH
 • CORTICOTROPIN
 • β LIPOTROPIN
 Met-ENKEPHALIN
 tyr-gly-gly-phe-met
 Leu ENKEPHALIN
 tyr-gly-gly-phe-leu
 β ENDORPHIN –
 31 aa has Met Enk
 in its sequence
 • can produce
   catatonia
 • like Morphine
 • dec Substance P
 • Short acting
   analgesics
 • Can produce total
   body analgesia
	Agonist/Antagonist
	 • Good analgesic
	 • Profuse sweating
	 NO resp depression
	 A resp stimulant
	
	 SIDE EFFECT
	 • Nausea, vomiting
	 • Euphoria
	 • Hallucinate
	 If give to a Morphine
	 addict – withdrawal
	 Naive – analgesia
	 Addicted – reversal
	
	 Derivatives:
	 BUTORPHANOL
	 BUPRENORPHINE
	 NALBUPHINE
	 (same as above)
		NOT an analgesic
		
		 • MEPERIDINE
		   derivative
		
		 EFFECTS
		 • Sedation
		 • Resp depression
		 • Constipation,
		   anti-diarrheal
		 • Dependence
		
		 ANTIDOTE
		 NALOXONE
			Very short acting
			 IV lasts 30 min
			 100 x more potent
			   than MORPHINE
			 Dose 0.1 mg
			 USE
			 Preoperatively or
			   intraoperatively
			
			 SIDE EFFECTS
			 • Muscle rigidity
			 • Interferes with
			   respiration
			 • Drug abuse

OXYMORPHONE [213]

- Analgesic
- Parent of NALOXONE by substituting C-C=C for the CH₃ on the N
- Do the same with MORPHINE, yields N-Allyl-Normorphine
- Bad side effects
- Hallucinations

CONTRAINDICATIONS OF MORPHINE-LIKE DRUGS

1. Asthmatics or resp problems
2. Hypothyroidism
3. Chronic adrenocortical insufficiency
4. Hepatic insufficiency

Causes:
Stupor, Coma, Apnea

MORPHINE ANTAGONISTS [214]

NALOXONE (Narcan®)
With pharm action alone:
- Antagonize all but Histamine release
- Admin: 0.4 mg doses
  @ 1 mg Naloxone: 30 mg Morphine
- Competitive inhibition
- Specific for opioid drugs
Antihallucinogenic
  – some psychotic patients

NALORPHINE (Nalline®)
Side Effect: hallucinations

LEVALLORPHAN (Lorfan®)

AMPHETAMINES
- Enhance CNS Analgesics
TRICYCLIC ANTIDEPRESSANTS
- Enhance MORPHINE

RECEPTORS	EFFECTS	AGONISTS	ANTAGONISTS
MU (μ)	Analgesia Resp depression Euphoria Physical depend	MORPHINE	NALOXONE PENTAZOCINE
KAPPA (κ)	Analgesia Resp depression Sedation Miosis	MORPHINE PENTAZOCINE	NALOXONE
SIGMA (ε)	Dysphoria Hallucinations Resp stimulation	PENTAZOCINE	NALOXONE
DELTA (δ)	??? Cardiovasc ? Analgesic ?	ENKEPHALINS	NALOXONE

PERIPHERAL ANALGESICS	SALICYLATES [215]	ANILINES [216]
ASPIRIN (ASA) Prototype • Narrow spectrum pain relief • D.O.C.: neuralgia, arthralgia, myalgia, cephalalgia	ACETYLSALICYLIC ACID (ASA, Aspirin) Na SALICYLATE Me SALICYLATE ECOTRIN®	ACETANILIDE PHENACETIN ACETAMINOPHEN (Tylenol®)
USES Pain, fever, inflammation, rheumatoid & osteo- arthritis • NOT for visceral pain	PROPERTIES Analgesic Antipyretic Antiinflammatory Uricosuric	PROPERTIES Analgesic Antipyretic
MECHANISM Inc pain threshold Site of tissue damage – PGE PGE: vasodilates, chemotaxis ASA prevents PGE release • Dec hyperalgesia • Acetylates cyclooxygenase • Dec PGE synthesis • Dec chemotaxis and damage ASA – Dec clotting (small dose) Dec Thromboxane (TXA) Acetylate platelet enzyme ASA – Dec PGI_2 (prostacyclin) PGI – Vasodilator – inhibits platelet aggregation (opposite of TXA) TXA affected >> PGI	ASA: Oral: Absorbed quickly, Low pKa = 3, Ion Trap • $T_{1/2}$ = 30 min • Volume dist – wide • Excreted by kidney as metabolites and ASA ASA – deacetylated to form sodium salicylate • Inhibits PG synthesis • NO tolerance develops • NO resp depression • Inc pain threshold peripherally • Dec incidence of transient ischemic attack • Dec incidence 2nd MI	ACETANILIDE & PHENACETIN • Toxicity • Bone marrow suppression ACETAMINOPHEN • Metabolite of first 2 • NO Reye's Syndrome Antipyretic – dec PGE in the hypothalamus • NOT antiinflammatory • NO dec PGE periph • NO gastric upset • NOT effective for arthritis • NOT uricosuric
OTHER PROPERTIES 1. Antipyretic – dec PGE in the hypothalamus 2. Antiinflammatory • dec PGE periph, dec vasodil and chemo-taxis 3. Anticoagulant • dec TXA • Prevents vasoconstriction • Interferes Vit K – factor synthesis 4. Antidiabetic • dec Insulin use 5. Blocks uterine contraction/ pain • dec PGF_{2a} • Interferes with labor 6. Closes patent ductus arteriosus prematurely • dec PGE_2 (5 & 6 Contraindication: pregnancy) 7. Reye's Syndrome • following a viral infection 8. Uricosuric – high doses (Uremic – low doses)	Na SALICYLATE • $T_{1/2}$ = 4 hrs • Metabolite of ASA Me SALICYLATE • 21 x more potent than ASA • Use: Sore muscles	TOXICITY • Liver poisoning TX Hemodialysis Hemoperfusion N-acetylcysteine

ACUTE ASPIRIN TOXICITY	
1. Tinnitus (early warning)	4. Loss of hearing
2. Nausea, vomiting	5. Headache
3. Gastritis	6. Confusion (salicylism)

7. Respiratory stim & depress – Stim: Tachypnea, results in: • resp alkalosis • loss of CO_2
8. Acid-Base imbalance • Metabolic acidosis
 • high ASA (acid)
 • dec oxidative phosphorylation • inc lactate
9. Electrolyte loss • inc excreted HCO_3^-, Na^+, K^+
10. Coma and death

PYRAZOLES [217]	ETHOPROPAZINE[218]	PROSTAGLANDIN ANALOGS [219]
ANTIPYRINE AMINOPYRINE PHENYLBUTAZONE	ANTIMUSCARINIC ANTI-Parkinson's	(New drugs) MISOPROSTOL (Cytotec®)

PYRAZOLES	ETHOPROPAZINE	PROSTAGLANDIN ANALOGS
ANTIPYRINE AMINOPYRINE • Toxicity associated	**PROPERTIES** •Analgesic (borderline) •Parasympatholytic •Antihistamine •Local Anesthetic	MISOPROSTOL • PGE$_1$ analog Mucoprotective • NO Gastritis • Inc mucous secretion

NSAID [220]
(Nonsteroidal Antiinflammatory Drugs)

USE
- Allergic to ASA
- Ulcers
- Liver problems

and thickness
- Dec gastric acidity
- Inc $NaHCO_3$ in duodenum
- Inc blood flow

PHENYLBUTAZONE
INDOMETHACIN
FENOPROFEN
IBUPROFEN
NAPROXEN
TOLMETIN

SIDE EFFECTS
Anticholinergic
Drowsiness, CNS Δ,
dizziness, confusion,
blurred vision, dry
mouth, Dec BP,
nausea, vomiting.

SIDE EFFECTS
- 40% Diarrhea
- Spotting, female
- Spontaneous abortions

PROPERTIES
Analgesic
Antipyretic
Antiinflammatory
(Uricosuric - mildly only Phenylbutazone)

TOXICITY
Seizures, tachycardia, agranulocytosis, pancytopenia, idiopathic thrombocytopenia purpura, jaundice.

SIDE EFFECTS / TOXICITY
- Gastric & Duodenal Ulcers
- Interstitial Nephritis (reversible)
- Anaphylaxis
- Death

TRICYCLIC ANTIDEPRESSANTS
• Enhances peripheral analgesics
POTENTIATION
• Central + Peripherally acting analgesics

PHENYLBUTAZONE
- Does NOT inhibit PGE synthesis
- Stabilizes lysosomal membranes
- Mild uricosuria
USE
1. Joint Pain, takes 2 – 3 days
2. Hodgkin's Disease
3. Pain assoc with: Bursitis, Muscles, Joints, Tendons
Toxicity bone marrow depression

GOUT Management [221]
1. Pain Relief (analgesia)
    COLCHICINE • Antimitotic, tubules
     • Dec chemotaxis
    INDOMETHACIN • Gout analgesic
     • Closes patent ductus • dec PGE$_2$
    NSAID: PHENYLBUTAZONE
     • Stabilizes lysosomal membrane, dec tissue destruction by WBC
2. Uricosuric • Inc excretion of uric acid
    PROBENECID • Dec antibiotic excreted
     • Dec uric acid absorption
    SULFINPYRAZONE • Dec PG synthesis
     • Prevents MI, antiarrhythmic
     • Blocks uric acid absorption
3. Dec uric acid synthesis
    ALLOPURINOL • Inhibits xanthine oxidase

OTHER NSAIDs :
(i.e. IBUPROFEN)
- DO inhibit PG synthesis
- Side Effects of ASA
  - Ulcers   • Nephritis
  - Liver damage • Delay of labor
- NOT uricosuric

4 CHEMOTHERAPY

76

CANCER CHEMOTHERAPY	NITROSOUREAS [290] BCNU (CARMUSTINE) CCNU (LOMUSTINE)	PROCARBAZINE [291]	L-ASPARAGINASE [292]	ETOPOSIDE (VP-16) [293]
MODE OF ACTION	Alkylating agents Inhibit DNA, RNA and protein synthesis Toxic if cell is dividing	DNA strand scission DNA and RNA synthesis is impaired Forms peroxide / formaldehyde	Deprives cells of asparagine	Not understood • Degradation of DNA • Inhibits nucleoside transport • Inhibits mito oxid-phos
RESISTANCE	? DNA repair • nondividing cells	DNA repair	L- ASPase inactivated by protease	NONE
USES	Limited use Malignant glioma Lipophilic Penetrates CNS	MOPP – Hodgkin's	ALL Therapy: L-ASPase + VX + PREDNISONE	Tx: resistant CA, Oat Cell CA, Testicular CA ETOPOSIDE + CISPLATIN + BLEOMYCIN
ADMINISTRATION ABSORPTION	IV: CARMUSTINE (BCNU) Oral: LOMUSTINE (CCNU)	Oral, parenteral Metabolized into AZO cmpd and H_2O_2	Oral: destroyed by acid IV or IM only	
DISTRIBUTION	Penetrates CNS	In Plasma and CSF / CNS		
EXCRETION	Kidney – urine	Kidney – urine		
SIDE EFFECTS	Delayed hematopoietic depression Renal toxicity	Nausea, vomiting, diarrhea, bone marrow suppression, Psych Disturbances • MAO Inhibitor Do NOT eat tyramine foods May develop nonlympho leukemia Disulfiram reaction – alcohol Mutagenic Teratogenic	Hypersensitivity Dec clotting factors Pancreatitis Neurotoxic	Bone marrow suppression

CANCER CHEMOTHERAPY	VINCRISTINE [273] (VX, ONCOVIN®)	VINBLASTINE [274] (VBL)
MODE OF ACTION	Vinca alkaloids Mitotic spindle poisons Combine with Tubulin – inhibit metaphase Phase specific – Mitosis Penetration into the cell – unknown	
RESISTANCE	• Increased efflux out of the Cell • Gene amplification of P-Glycoprotein Also resistant to: DOXORUBICIN ACTINOMYCIN D	
USES	<u>MOPP</u> VX: Acute LØ leukemia (ALL) Ewing's sarcoma Hodgkin's disease Wilm's tumor	<u>ABVD</u> VBL: Testicular tumors • with CISPLASTIN • with BLEOMYCIN CHORIOCARCINOMA Hodgkin's disease
ADMINISTRATION ABSORPTION	IV bolus injection • Inc uric acid (hyperuricemia) • Give ALLOPURINOL – xanthine oxidase inhibitor	
DISTRIBUTION	Concentrated in the liver	
EXCRETION	In bile → feces Hepatic function impaired – modify dose	
SIDE EFFECTS	VX: Paralytic ileus Phlebitis / Cellulitis Nausea, vomiting Diarrhea Alopecia Neurotoxic • Ataxia • Peripheral neuropathy Microtubule lesions Inc ADH – hydrate well	VBL: Paralytic ileus Phlebitis / Cellulitis Nausea, vomiting Diarrhea Alopecia Bone marrow suppression (myelosuppression)

HORMONES		AMINO [277]	
PREDNISONE [275]	ESTROGEN [276]	GLUTETHIMIDE	TAMOXIFEN [278]
Antiinflammatory due to: • Cushing's syndrome • Lymphocytopenia Dec LØ mass by bind recptr protein • Nucleus → DNA → Proteins	Antagonizes effect of male sex hormone Physiologic (NOT Cytotoxic)	Inhibits PREGNENOLONE • Inhibits aromatic Rxn in formation of sex hormones • P_{450} Inducer D.O. 2nd Choice	Related to DES • Antiestrogen • Antiprogesterone Acts only on tissue with EST or PROG receptors • Forms a complex with receptors – inactive
Rodent Model: – Dec # or absent receptors Affinity of receptors NOT correlated with resistance			ESTROGEN • Better affinity for receptor • Works best in postmenopause Dec biofeedback to pituitary to stim FSH production
Lymphoma Leukemia – ALL MOPP • Hodgkin's therapy • NonHodgkin's		Prostatic Cancer 1. GB 2. LHRH (9 aa) • Agonist/antagonist • Leuprolide Greater potency than LHRH Dec gonadotropin secretion	Breast cancer palliative Endometrial cancer
Oral	Oral		Oral
			Liver Metabolism Bile → Feces
Hyper adrenal cortisolism Mental aberrations Gastric ulcers		Dizziness Ataxia Lethargy **HODGKIN'S DISEASE THERAPY** 1. MOPP • MECHLORETHAMINE • ONCOVIN (VINCRISTINE) • PREDNISONE & PROCARBAZINE 2. ABVD • ADRIAMYCIN • BLEOMYCIN • VINBLASTINE • DACARBAZINE	Nausea, vomiting vaginal bleeding and discharge Hot flashes Rash If metastasized to bone → Pain Teratogenic in experimental animals

CANCER CHEMOTHERAPY	ANTIBIOTICS – Cell Cycle Specific		
	ACTINOMYCIN D (DACTINOMYCIN) [279]	DOXORUBICIN (ADRIAMYCIN®) DAUNORUBICIN [280]	BLEOMYCIN [281]

MODE OF ACTION	Isolated from *Streptomyces*
	 • Intercalates into DNA
	 • Inhib DNA depend RNA Polymerase
	 • Inc [ ] – Dec DNA synthesis
	 • DNA scission
	   • by O radical
		Intercalates DNA
		 • S Phase specific
		 P_{450} Reductase →
		   Q radical
		 Quinone rd → O rd
		 • Strand Scission
		 Binds the cell memb
		 • Δ Transport of
		   Phos– Inositol
			A Peptide with Cu^{++}
			 Reacts with Fe^{++}
			 Fe-Cu DNA complex
			 • Oxid Chromosome
			 • G_2 Phase

RESISTANCE	P-Glycoprotein • Inc efflux Inc DNA repair	P Glyco-Protein • Inc efflux Dec uptake Dec P_{450} reductase DNA repair	Unknown

USES	Wilm's Tumor
	 Choriocarcinoma
	 Soft-tissue
	   Sarcoma
		DOXORUBICIN
		 • ALL – solid tumor
		 • Breast, Lung,
		   Lymph
		 • Hodgkin's
		 DAUNORUBICIN
		 – AML
			Testicular CA
			 • with VBL +
			   ETOPOSIDE

ADMINISTRATION	IV – Conc in liver	IV – Widely
		   distributed
			IM, IV, SQ
			 Metabolized by a
			   hydroxylase
			 Dec hydroxylase in
			   lung & skin, more
			   susceptible
			 Inc hydroxylase
			   Sarcoma resistant

DISTRIBUTION		Widely distributed Penetrates CNS	
EXCRETION	Parenteral cmpd & metabs excreted in the bile	Excreted in Bile Some into urine - red Give TOCOPHEROL	Kidney: Glomerular filtrate, Renal failure: Dec dose
SIDE EFFECTS	Bone marrow depression • Nausea, vomiting, diarrhea, alopecia, stomatitis, extravasation problem, radiation sensitivity	Toxic: Tissues with low level of superox dismutase • Cardiotoxic • Tissue necrosis • Bone marrow depr stomatitis, alopecia, GI disturbances	Mucocutaneous hyperpigmentation Limiting toxicity • Pulmonary fibrosis • Dose related > 400 mg/ml Alopecia <u>NO Marrow Depres</u>

| ALKYLATING AGENTS | | |
MECHLORETHAMINE [282]	CYCLOPHOSPHAMIDE [283]	CISPLATIN [284]

Nitrogen Mustard
• Alkylate N(7) guanine
• Depurination
  Nicks DNA, Breaks
• Cross link chain
• Miscoding
Proliferating cells more
  sensitive
Rapid onset
	Nitrogen Mustard
	• Hydroxylation by P_{450} to
	  PHOSPHORAMIDE
	  MUSTARD
	  (+) ACROLEIN
	Both cytotoxic
		$$NH_3 \diagdown \; Cl^-$$ $$Pt^{++}$$ $$NH_3 \diagup \; Cl^-$$
		
		$Cl^- > OH^-$, Exchanged
		Binds DNA
		Intrastrand bridge
		Cross link
		Inhibits RNA synthesis (G_1, S)

DNA repair Dec permeability	DNA repair Dec permeability	DNA repair
Hodgkin's MOPP Solid tumors	Burkitt's lymphoma Breast cancer Multiple sclerosis Myasthenia Rheumatoid arthritis Nephrotic syndrome	Testicle cancer • with VBL (+) BLEOMYCIN Ovarian cancer (+) DOXORUBICIN Bladder cancer

Choline uptake system
• Takes drug up
IV
• Severe tissue damage if
  extravasation
	Oral (unusual – Mustard)
	Liver metabolism
	Phosphoramide mustard
	  distributed
		IV • in Saline
		• Stabilizes Cl
		• 90% PPB

		Does NOT penetrate CNS/CSF Concentrated: Liver, Ovary, Kidney, GI
	Feces Urine	Renal excretion Ca^{++} Loss Mg^{++} Loss

Severe vomiting ,
Herpes zoster
• Latent, reappears
Severe marrow depression
GI toxicity
Mutagenic
Teratogenic
	Nausea, vomiting, diarrhea
	Hemorrhagic cystitis
	(give Na^+ 2- Mercaptoethane
	  Sulfonate)
	Inc ADH (like VX)
	Amenorrhea, testicle
	  atrophy, sterility,
	Immunosuppress, Dec bile
		Vomit 100% (severe)
		Nephrotoxic, Ototoxic
		• Hearing loss • tinnitus
		Hypersensitive
		• Rash/Anaphylactic
		Slightly neurotoxic
		• Paresthesia
		Slight marrow suppression

CANCER CHEMOTHERAPY	METHOTREXATE [285]	6-MERCAPTOPURINE (6-MP) [286]
MODE OF ACTION Cell cycle specific Antimetabolites (S Phase)	Antifolate Dec DNA and RNA Cell death DHF $-/\rightarrow$ THF Inhibits DHF reductase N^5 Formyl THF • Thymidylic acid • Purines N^{5-10} Methyl THF • Pyrimidine	Converts to 6-MP ribose-P HGPRTase – Salvage path Catalyzes the addition of ribose phosphate Inhibits 1st Step *de novo* purine synthesis Incorporated into DNA
RESISTANCE	Gene amplification • Inc DHF reductase Dec affinity of MTX for DHF Reduc P-Glycoprotein • Inc Efflux Dec Permeability Inc Thymidylate Syntase	Inability to biotransform due to Dec protease (Lesch – Nyhan syndrome) Inc metabolism to thiouric acid
USES	ALL (maintenance) Choriocarcinoma Breast CA, Psoriasis, Osteogenic sarcoma • Very high dose for 24 hrs + Folinic acid	Maintain ALL remission
ADMINISTRATION ABSORPTION	Oral, IM, IV, IT Taken up by mostly active transport Diffusion at high conc Converts to polyglutamates • Stays in the cell	Oral • Preferred • Well absorbed Liver Metab $\rightarrow$ Thiourate Catalyzed by xanthine oxidase ALLOPURINOL inhibits xanth oxidase – Dec dose
DISTRIBUTION	Does NOT cross BBB/CNS Plasma protein bound • Can be displaced by TETRACYCLINE, ASPIRIN, CHLORAMPHENICOL MTX enters cells via a special transport system, same as cofactors for polyglutamate	
EXCRETION	Hydroxylated • Some activity • Less soluble • High [ ] $\rightarrow$ Crystalluria	
SIDE EFFECTS	Nausea, vomiting, diarrhea, stomatitis, alopecia, erythema – rash, urticaria megaloblastic anemia, bone marrow suppress (Give folinic acid + LEUCOVORIN®) Hepatic fibrosis IT: Headache, Seizures	Nausea, vomiting, diarrhea Thrombocytopenia Long Tx $\rightarrow$ Bile stasis Cholangiolitic hepatitis esp with DOXORUBICIN

6-THIOGUANINE (6-TG) [287]	5-FLUOROURACIL (5-FU) [288]	CYTARABINE (ARA-C) [289]
Converts to nucleotide Inhibits purine synthesis at feedback inhibitor sites Inhibits phosphorylation of dGMP → dGDP Incorporated into DNA	5 FU-dUMP competes for thymidylate synthase • Dec synthesis DNA Pyrimidine antagonist	Pyrimidine antagonist Converts to nucleotide Inhibits DNA synth (Polymerase) Inhibits CDP → dCDP Incorp DNA/RNA
	Dec deoxynucleotides Dec affinity for thymidylate synthase Inc amount natural Substrate dUMP	Dec production of abnormal nucleotide Dec affinity for DNA polymerase Inc dCTP Inc methylation of ARA-C → ARA-U
AML Therapy: 6-TG + ARA-C + DAUNORUBICIN	Solid tumors: • Colon cancer • Breast cancer • Ovarian cancer • Pancreatic cancer • Gastric cancer	AML therapy 6-TP + ARA-C + DAUNORUBRICIN
Oral (ALLOPURINOL does NOT help)	Topical Basal cell cancer IV	NOT effective oral • Forms ARA-U in the intestine Parenterally – IV
	Penetrates well including CNS	Throughout body NOT in CNS
	Bile – Feces	Kidney – urine
(Same as 6-MP) Nausea, vomiting, diarrhea, thrombocytopenia Long Tx → Bile stasis Cholangiolitic hepatitis esp with DOXORUBICIN	Nausea, vomiting, diarrhea, Bone marrow suppression, Ulcers: Oral & GI, Anorexia, Acute cerebellar syndrome • Nystagmus • Slurred speech • Ataxia	Nausea, vomiting Diarrhea Alopecia Potent myelosuppression (Bone marrow suppression) Hepatic dysfunction

5 ENDOCRINE

DIABETES INSULIN [345]	REGULAR (CRYSTALLINE)	ISOPHANE, NPH (Neutral Protamine H)	INSULIN ZINC SUSP (LENTE)	PROTAMINE ZINC INSULIN (PZI)	INSULIN ZINC SUSP (ULTRALENTE)
TYPE	Rapid acting IV – only one	Delayed onset Longer duration Intermediate acting IM or SQ	Delayed onset Longer duration Intermediate acting IM or SQ	Long onset Long duration Long acting IM or SQ	Long onset Long duration Long acting IM or SQ
USE	Diabetic emergency Hyperglycemic shock Peak = ½ to 3 hr $T_{1/2}$ = 5 – 7 hr	Most commonly used Peak = 8 – 12 hr $T_{1/2}$ = 18 – 24 hr	Peak = 8 – 12 hr $T_{1/2}$ = 8 – 24 hr	Peak = 8 – 16 hr $T_{1/2}$ = 24 – 36 hr	Peak = 8 – 16 hr $T_{1/2}$ = 24 – 36 hr

SIDE EFFECTS	1. HYPOGLYCEMIA
	Young patient:
	Autonomic hyperactivity
	• Symp: Tachycardia
	  Palpitations
	  Sweating
	• Parasymp: Nausea
	  Hunger
	• Coma and death
		2. HYPOGLYCEMIA
		Elderly patient
		• Mental confusion
		• Convulsions
		• Coma and death
		Tx: Insulin Induced hypoglycemia
		• Oral glucose
		• IV glucose (50%)
		• IM / SQ glucagon
				3. INSULIN ALLERGY
				• Immediate Type I
				  Local or systemic
				  Urticaria (hives)
				  Anaphylaxis – severe
				• Immune Complex
				  Type III
				  Arthus-like reaction
				  (local)
					4. LIPOATROPHY
					Atrophy of subcutaneous
					fatty tissue at site of
					injection
					
					5. Other
					• Paresthesia
					• Sweating

GENERAL	Inc glucose uptake into tissue
	Dec blood glucose level
	Dec gluconeogenesis
	
	Prepared in 40 – 100 std vials
	Potency in USP
	From pig and cow
		FACTORS AFFECTING DOSE
		1. Exercise – Dec dose
		  Acts like insulin
		2. Stress – Inc dose
		  emotional, infection, allergy, fever
		3. Pregnancy – Inc dose
		4. Drugs – Inc dose
		  Corticosteroids (GC)
		  Oral contraceptives (EST)
		  Thiazides
				CONTRAINDICATED
				Overeat
				Overdose
				Exercise
				Hormone drugs
				
				INDICATED FOR
				IDDM	

HYPOTHALAMIC PITUITARY

PHYSIOLOGICAL EFFECTS
• Endogenous level
• Normal

PHARMACOLOGICAL EFFECTS
• Exogenous (reaction)
• Greater levels

FOUR CLASSES
1. AMINES • Catecholamine
2. IODOTHYRONINES • Thyroid hormones
3. PEPTIDES
• Water soluble
• Surface receptor
• Conformational Δ
• Antagonist binds rcptr
4. STEROIDS
• Plasma protein for transport
• Lipid Soluble
• Cytoplasmic receptors
• Antagonist binds rcptr

ANTERIOR PITUITARY
• Hypothalamo-hypo-physeal portal circulation

POSTERIOR PITUITARY
• Intracellular transport inside of neurons

ANTERIOR PITUITARY HORMONES

ACTH [294]	PROLACTIN [295]	GROWTH HORMONE [296]	FSH/LH [297]
CRF (+) Hypothalamus CORTISOL (-) Feedback	PRH (+) Hypothalamus PIF (-) Hypothalamus Dopamine (DA)	GRH (+) Hypothalamus SOMATOSTATIN (-)	GnRH (+)
Peptide hormone Inc conversion of Cholesterol → Pregnenolone Rate limiting step and where AMINOGLU-TETHEMIDE inhibits	Controls lactation • After birth, Sharp Dec in EST & PROG Breast feed – Stim lactation • Inhibits ovulation, 6 – 9 months	Acts on LIVER to produce → Somatomedins • Linear body growth • Inc the metabolic rate of all body tissues	GnRH pulsatile release HIGH Conc GnRH • Down regulate receptors • Dec LH and FSH
Inc corticosteroids: glucocorticoids, mineralo-corticoids, androgens Diagnostic Use Only NOT used for replacement Tx		GH only used to treat hypopituitary dwarfism See BROMOCRIPTINE in the Tx of acromegaly below	**MALE** LH • Stim TEST synthesis • Stim sperm production FSH • Inc sertoli function • Sperm production **FEMALE** LH • Stim EST & PROG • Surge → ovulation FSH • Follicle maturation before ovulation

TSH [298]
TRH (+)
• Thyroxine
• T_3 & T_4

POSTERIOR PITUITARY HORMONES

OXYTOCIN [299]	VASOPRESSIN [ADH (Antidiuretic Hormone)] [300]	DESOMPRESSIN [301]
Smooth muscle contraction • Stimulates milk secretion / ejection • Stimulates uterine contractions	**ADMIN** IV or nasal (NOT oral) Responds to: Inc plasma Osm, Dec BP, Dec blood vol Deficiency = DI (diabetes insipidus) High Conc → Constricts splanchnics ∴ Esophageal varices & DI Inc H_2O reabsorption in collecting ducts Inhibited by alcohol	Vasopressin analog Admin: nasal Advantage: long duration Inc H_2O reabsorption

THERAPEUTIC PHARMACOLOGY

BROMOCRIPTINE [302]	HMG [303]	HCG [304]	LEUPROLIDE [305]	GONADORELIN [306]
DOPAMINE AGONIST Ergot alkaloid	Human Menopausal Gonadotropin	Human Chorionic Gonadotropin	GnRH agonist	GnRH analog
Dec PROLACTIN	Contains LH + FSH	LH analog	Long acting agonist	NOT used because requires infusion pump for many days or weeks
• Directly on PIH receptor in anterior pituitary	Post menopausal urine	Pregnant mother's urine	Initial Inc in LH/FSH Down regulates GnRH receptors	
• Inc DA levels in hypothalamus	**Rx**	Placental hormone	Dec LH & FSH (2° Dec in estrogens)	
USES	Infertility	**Rx**		
1. Mother NOT breast feeding	**SIDE EFFECT**	Infertility	**SIDE EFFECTS**	
• Dec Prolactin	Multiple births		• Headaches	
• Helps "Dry Up"			• Dry vagina	
• Allows ovulation			• Hot flashes	
2. Hyperprolactinemia			**Rx**	
→ Amenorrhea – return of cycle			1. Endometriosis	
			2. Precocious puberty	
GROWTH HORMONE			3. Infertility	
• Normal				
• Inc GH secretion				
• Acromegaly				
• BROMO will cause Dec GH secretion				

SIDE EFFECTS
Anorexia, nausea, vomiting, constipation, postural hypotension, digital vasospasm, arrhythmias, confusion, hallucination, headache, nasal congestion, pulmonary infiltration, tender hands & feet, alcohol intolerance

---

INFERTILITY THERAPY
HYPOTHALAMIC AMENORRHEA

1. HMG
   - (LH and FSH) FSH will cause follicles to mature
   - Often multiple births
2. LEUPROLIDE
   - Depresses LH and FSH, do NOT get LH surge
   - Follicles do NOT ovulate before they are mature
3. HCG
   - Use last, LH activity will stimulate ovulation

ADRENAL STEROIDS

Cholesterol derivatives
<u>CORTICOSTEROIDS</u> [307]
1. GLUCOCORTICOIDS (GC)
   - Glycogen storage
   - Δ blood glucose levels • 1° cortisol
2. MINERALOCORTICOIDS (MC)
   - Na^+ / water retention (kidney)
   - 1° aldosterone
Overlap in function between the
corticosteroids

<u>KINETICS</u>
1. Rapid Absorption
2. Protein bound 85% α_2 globulin
   10% albumin   5% free → Pharm effect
3. Metabolized – liver
4. Excreted – kidney, 17-ketosteroids

<u>GLUCOCORTICOIDS</u> (GC)
ACTH-mediated
Cholesterol → Pregnenolone
NOT stored, synthesized on demand
Diffuse through membrane → Cyto R
  → Nucleus → Δ Transcript / Translation

<u>CONTROL</u>
1. CRF • Hypothalamus → Ant Pituitary
2. ACTH • Ant Pit → Adrenal cortex
3. Cortisol • Peripheral effect • Feedback
   Inhibition at both Hypothal and Ant Pit
   (+) Feedback – low levels
   (-) Feedback – high levels
<u>Circadian Rhythm</u> • Diurnal
   - Peak – when waking up
   - Trough – when sleeping

<u>EFFECTS</u>
A. ANTIINFLAMMATORY
   1. Dec Inflammation and swelling
   2. Inhib arachidonic acid synthesis
   3. Inhibit phospholipase A_2
      → Dec leukotrienes, Dec prostaglandins
   4. Dec capillary permeability
   - Dec diapedesis • Inhib MØ, LØ, EØ, BØ
   - Dec interleukin • Dec PMN chemotaxis
   5. Inhibits histamine release (BØ)
   6. Dec lysosomal enzyme releases
      Stabilizes lysosomal membrane
   7. Inhibits LØ, Dec Ab – lymphatic atrophy

B. Δ PROTEIN METABOLISM
   1. Dec protein synthesis
   2. Inc catabolism (breakdown)
   3. (-) Nitrogen balance
   4. Muscle wasting
   5. Osteoporosis

C. Δ CARBOHYDRATE METABOLISM
Carbo sparing effect – anti-insulin
1. Inc blood glucose
2. Inc gluconeogenesis
3. Inc glycogenesis
4. Block glu transport into muscle and
   adipose
Hyperglycemic / Insulin resistant

D. LIPID METABOLISM INCREASED
Low levels – lipolytic
High levels – lipogenesis
Insulin release is stimulated
Fat redistribution
   - Moon Face, Buffalo Hump

E. HYPOKALEMIC Alkalosis
   2° Inc Na^+ / water retention
   Inc K^+, H^+, Ca^{++} excretion
   Ca^{++} loss → bone loss

<u>USES</u>
1. Substitution therapy
   a. Addison's disease
   b. Adrenogenital hyperplasia
2. Inflammation suppression
   a. Rheumatoid arthritis
   b. SLE   d. Asthma
   c. Urticaria   e. Edema
3. Immunosuppression
   a. Graft rejection
   b. Idiopathic thrombocytopenic purpura

<u>SIDE EFFECTS</u> Dose-related
1. PSYCHIATRIC REACTION • Euphoria,
   Psychotic, paranoid, depression
2. PEPTIC ULCERS
   a. Inc pepsin and HCl
   b. Dec gastric mucosa cell proliferation
3. HYPERTENSION
   Na^+ and water retention   2° MC effect
4. DIABETES MELLITUS
   a. Hyperglycemia
   b. Causes insulin resistance
5. CATARACTS
   - Post subcapsular • Irreversible
6. ALLERGIES
7. SUPPRESS HYP–PIT–ADR AXIS
8. MYOPATHY
9. OSTEOPOROSIS
   - Dec Ca^{++} • Bone loss
10. DEC COLLAGEN • Inhib fibroblasts
    - Weak CT, thin skin, . . .
11. PREDISPOSED TO INFECTION

ADRENAL STEROIDS			
GLUCOCORTICOID	Antiinflammatory	Na⁺ Retention	

GLUCOCORTICOID	Antiinflammatory	Na⁺ Retention	
Short Acting GC			
CORTISONE	0.8	0.8	
CORTISOL	1.0	1.0	
Intermediate GC			
PREDNISONE	4	0.8	
PREDNISOLONE	4	0.8	
METHYL PREDNISOLONE	5	0.5	
TRIAMCINOLONE	5	0.0	
Long Acting GC			
DEXAMETHASONE	25	0.0	Tx: Asthma
BETAMETHASONE	25	0.0	
MINERALOCORTICOID			
Short Acting MC			
ALDOSTERONE	0.1	500	Tx: Adrenal
FLUDROCORTISONE	10.0	125	Insuffic

CONTRAINDICATIONS (glucocorticoids)
1. Pregnancy and long-acting GC
        DEXAMETHASONE – teratogenic
2. Growing children • 2 to 4 yrs and puberty – growing
                • Suppresses GH secretion – Dec bone growth
                (Use ACTH instead. but ACTH is not as effective as GC)
3. Drug interactions
                a. Increase INSULIN
                b. PHENOBARBITAL • Inc the metabolism of GC
                c. Inc DIGOXIN toxicity because hypokalemia → arrhythmia

ANTAGONISTS of corticosteroids [308]

1. SPIRONOLACTONE
  • K⁺ Sparing diuretic • Inc Na⁺ & H_2O excretion
  • Competitive inhibitor of aldosterone receptor • Block MC effects of the aldosterone
2. MITOTANE
  • Very potent • Treat adrenal cancer • Destroys the adrenal cortex at very high doses
3. AMINOGLUTETHIMIDE
  • Block GC synthesis (1st Step)
  • Inhibits all adrenal hormone synthesis at cholesterol → pregnenolone
  • Tx: adrenal malignancy (GC Excess)
4. METYRAPONE
  • Blocks cortisol synthesis only – inhibits 11 OHase (deoxycortisol –/→ cortisol)
  • Tx: Cushing's disease

> Primary control of Cortisol is by ACTH
> (with a minor effect by Angiotensin II)
>
> Primary control of Aldosterone
> is by Angiotensin II
> (with a minor effect by ACTH)

ADRENAL STEROIDS	GLUCOCORTICOIDS [309]	MINERALO- CORTICOIDS [310]	DEXAMETHASONE BETAMETHASONE [311]	TRIAMCINOLONE [312]	FLUDROCORTISONE [313]
	CORTISOL	ALDOSTERONE	Synthetic CORTISOL		Synthetic ALDOSTERONE
ADMINISTRATION	$T_{1/2}$ = 90 min, Topical		IV, PO, IM		
EFFECTS	Antiinflammatory Inhibit phospholipase A_2 • Dec PG • Dec LT • Dec LPX Negative nitrogen balance Inc blood glucose • Dec utilization • Inc gluconeogenesis • Inc glycogen Lipolytic • Dec fat synthesis Fat deposition • at high doses (insulin) Minor mineralocorticoid	Inc water retention Inc Na⁺ retention Inc K⁺ excretion		Glucocorticoid with NO mineralocorticoid action	
SIDE EFFECTS		Hypokalemic alkalosis	Psychiatric, peptic ulcer, HT, cataracts, myelopathy, osteoporosis, Hyp-Pit axis suppression DEXAMETH – teratogenic		
CONTRAINDICATED			Diabetes, pregnancy, digoxin, phenobarbital		
TREATMENT			Addison's, SLE, asthma, congenital adrenal hyperplasia, rheumatoid arthritis, thrombocytopenic purpura, graft rejection	Rheumatoid arthritis, systemic lupus erythematosus	Adrenal insufficiency

ADRENAL ANTAGONISTS	SPIRONOLACTONE [314]	MITOTANE [315]	AMINOGLUTETHIMIDE [316]	METOPIRONE [317] (Metyrapone®)
MECHANISM	Competitive inhibitor of aldosterone Reversibly binds aldosterone receptors		Competitively inhibits the enzyme Desmolase in the first step in the synthesis of adrenal hormones: Cholesterol → Pregnenolone	Inhibits 11 - β hydroxylase
EFFECT	K^+ sparing diuretic Blocks Na^+ reabsorption Inc H_2O excretion	Dec or blocks all adrenal hormone synthesis Large doses can destroy the adrenal gland	Inhibits all adrenal hormone synthesis	Blocks cortisol synthesis Inc mineralocorticoids
TOXICITY	Hypertension	Adrenal carcinoma	Adrenal Carcinoma + Hypersecretion	Cushing's Disease

ANDROGENS [318]	ANABOLIC STEROIDS [319]

ANDROGENS [318]

SYNTHESIS
MALE: 10% adrenal cortex 90% testis
FEMALE: adrenal cortex, ovaries, peripheral
conversion

5α-reductase
TESTOSTERONE → D-HT
NUCLEAR RECEPTOR

MALE
1. *In utero* • Sex development
2. Puberty • 2° sex characteristics • Sperm production
 • 30% Inc bone growth • Closes epiphyseal plates
3. Adult • Maintain sperm production
 • Libido • Anabolic (Inc mass)

FEMALE
1. TEST is the EST precursor
2. Puberty • 2° sex, hair • Growth spurts
3. Adult – libido

INDICATIONS
1. 1° replacement therapy
2. Anemia • High doses will stimulate
 Hb and RBC production
3. Osteoporosis • Unproven
 • Inc Ca++ deposition (EST is used)
4. Breast Cancer • EST-dependent CA
 • by (-) feedback • Suppresses GnRH
 → Dec LH/FSH → Dec EST • Anti-EST now used
5. Endometriosis • (DANAZOL is the D.O.C.)
6. Fibrocystic breast disease
7. Angioneurotic edema • Hereditary, rare
 • Local edema: face, neck, hands, feet

PHARMACOLOGIC ANDROGENS:
1. Natural testosterone
 • NOT administered orally (1st pass)
 • Short acting
2. Testosterone esters:
 TESTOSTERONE PROPIONATE
 TESTOSTERONE ENANTHATE
 TESTOSTERONE CYPIONATE
 • NOT administered orally
 • Longer acting (Dec metabolism)
3. Synthetic: METHYLTESTOSTERONE
 FLUOXYMESTERONE
 • Methyl at carbon 17 (hepatotoxic)
 • Oral administration • Longest duration

SIDE EFFECTS
1. FEMALE:
 • Masculinization • Dec breast size
 • Inc body hair
 • Inc sebaceous gland activity (Acne)
2. MALE:
 • Feminization
 • Gynecomastia (high doses)
 • Peripheral conversion to EST in liver and adipose
 • Dec spermatogenesis because Dec LH and FSH
3. Liver disorder • Methyl at C17
 • Monitor enzyme levels
4. Hepatocellular Carcinoma ? (Me C17)

PROGESTERONE, ESTROGEN and ANDROGEN
 activity may overlap

ANABOLIC STEROIDS [319]

STANOZOLOL
NANDROLONES
OXYMETHOLONE
OXANDROLONE
FLUOXYMESTERONE
DROMOSTANOLONE
Δ Androgen properties
Inc Body mass – 60 to 100 lbs / yr
 • Only in conditioned athletes
 • Does NOT affect non-exercisers

INDICATIONS NONE
 • But still listed for angioneurotic edema
 (DANAZOL is D.O.C.)
 • Used in the past to Tx • Burn victims
 • Undernourished

SIDE EFFECTS
Same as androgens but exaggerated
 because of abuse, 10 – 100 times dose
1. FEMALE • Masculinize
2. MALE • Feminize • Dec sperm produced
 • Dec steroid synthesis
3. Liver damage
4. Hepatocellular CA
5. Cholestatic jaundice
6. Anabolic: Inc protein synth → Inc mass
7. Na+ & H₂0 retention
8. Aggressive, psychotic behavior
Most have methyl at C17, causing liver
 toxicity

ANDROGEN	TESTOSTERONE [320]	DANAZOL [321]	DERIVATIVES [322]	SYNTHETIC [323]	ANABOLIC STEROIDS [324]
DURATION	Short		Longer	Longest	
ROUTE	IV, IM		IV, IM	Oral	
EFFECTS	Converted to DHT Differentiates male sex development • Wolffian • Stimulates 2° sex • Initiate sperm production • Growth & libido • Stimulate Hb synthesis • Inc Ca++ deposit – bone • Feedback inhib hypoth 1st pass • Can't give orally Masculinize women Feminize men	NOT an androgen Binds receptors of: • ANDROGEN • PROGESTERONE • Glucocorticoid (-) Feedback on hypothalamus → Dec GnRh → Dec LH/FSH Dec EST	Testosterone derivatives • Testost Propionate • Testost Enanthate • Testost Cypionate	Methyl Testosterone Fluroxymesterone C17 - Methyl SIDE EFFECTS • Liver disease • Jaundice • Cancer	STANOZOLOL. SIDE EFFECTS • Liver disease • Aggressive behavior
	Replacement Tx Anemia Osteoporosis Breast CA Endometriosis	Endometriosis Fibrocystic breast Breast CA Angioneurotic edema			Angioneurotic edema

ESTROGENS [325]
ANTIFERTILITY AGENTS

ESTROGENS • Induce estrus
PROGESTINS • Formation of secretory
  endometrium

SYNTHESIS
From Androgens
1. Testosterone → Estradiol (ovary)
2. Estradiol → Estriol (liver)
  (1° source of estriol)
3. Δ4 • Androstenedione → Estrone (liver)

ACTIONS
1. PUBERTY: FEMALE 2° SEX
 • Stim release of GH (Growth Hormone)
 • Closes epiphyseal plate
2. DEVELOPS ENDOMETRIAL LINING
  During the menstrual cycle
3. MENSTRUAL CYCLE
a. Many follicles mature /grow (FSH)
b. One will develop more
  → 1° follicle – ovulates
 • Other follicles regress
c. 1° Follicle • synthesizes ESTROGEN
 • Controlled by LH
 • EST peak in 1st half of cycle
d. EST → Endometrium proliferates
  Prepares uterus for implantation
e. Before ovulation – sharp Dec EST
f. Then massive Inc LH surge
  from Ant Pit → ovulation
g. Corpus luteum left behind
h. CL • Synthesizes PROGESTINS
    • Inc PROG 2nd half cycle
i. PROG • 1° Effect Δ endometrium
  proliferating → secreting endometrium
 • Inc glycogen, glandular tissue
 • Stabilizes endometrium
j. If implantation occurs
 • CL – PROG synthesis continues until
  placenta develops and takes over
  PROG synthesis
k. NO implantation
  CL degenerates • Dec PROG
  Loss of stabilizing effect on endometrium
  → shed, menses
4. ANTAGONIZES PTH
 • Slows bone resorption (Dec breakdown)
 • Does NOT restore bone
5. Δ LIPOPROTEINS
 • Dec LDL
 • Inc HDL

INDICATIONS
1. REPLACEMENT THERAPY
  (Must give with PROGESTIN)
2. POST-MENOPAUSAL Tx
 • Ovaries Dec synthesis of ESTROGEN
 • Symptoms: Hot flashes, atrophic
  vaginitis, anxiety, Inc sweating
3. OSTEOPOROSIS
 • Could be life-threatening
 • Greatest risk: Family history
4. ANDROGEN-DEPENDENT TUMORS
 • Tx: Prostatic CA
 • Exerts feedback inhibit - hypothalamus
 • Dec GnRH → Dec LH/FSH
  → Dec androgen
5. ORAL CONTRACEPTIVES
  Effectively prevents pregnancy
a. Inhibits ovulation
b. Makes endometrium inappropriate
  for implantation
c. Dec LH, FSH, PROG, ESTRADIOL
  Feedback inhibition
6. ESTROGEN
 • NEVER alone
 • Always with PROGESTIN

PHARMACOKINETICS
All do the same thing
Differ only by absorption, metabolism
 and duration
All effective orally
1. Natural esters
  ESTRADIOL • Most abundant and potent
 • Prototype, replacement therapy
 • Significant absorption
 • Signif 1st pass liver metabolism
  Need high doses
ESTRIOL
ESTRONE
2. Conjugated EST
 • Sulfate conjugates
 • Urine of pregnant horses
 • Dec metab, Inc duration
3. EST esters
 • Dec Metab, Inc duration
4. Synthetic steroidal EST
ETHINYL ESTRADIOL
MESTRANOL
 • In oral contraceptives (OC)
 • Slowest metabolism
 • Longest duration

ESTROGENS [326]
ANTIFERTILITY AGENTS

5. Nonsteroidal
DIETHYLSTIBESTROL (DES)
CHLOROTRIANISENE
ETHINYL ESTRADIOL
• Good absorption
• NO 1st pass metabolism
• Does NOT look like EST, but can bind
  EST receptors
• Agonists – EST activity

SIDE EFFECTS
Minor: Nausea, headache, post
menopausal bleeding, tender breasts,
Δ plasma proteins

Major:

1. FLUID RETENTION
• Stim hepatic angiotensinogen
→ Inc angiotensin II
→ Stimulate aldosterone
→ Na+ / Water retention

2. HYPERTENSION
• Assoc with oral contraceptives
  (NOT with replacement therapy)
• 30% Inc mild hypertension

3. GALL BLADDER DISEASE (GB)
• Assoc with post menopausal
  replacement therapy
• Significant 1st pass effect, because
  larger dose required
  → Inc GB disease
• non oral ESTRADIOL
  NO GB disease
• Transdermal patch low dose
  NO GB disease

4. CLOTTING DISORDERS
Inc 2 – 3 times risk of
• Thromboembolic disease
• Pulmonary emboli
• Strokes
EST Stimulates Inc synthesis of
factors II, VII, X and fibrinogen
• Assoc with oral high dose

5. MYOCARDIAL INFARCTION (MI)
Slight Inc risk MI
Only if already high risk:
     smoke, obese, IDDM

CONTRAINDICATED
1. Smoking women > 35 yrs
   Non smoking women > 40 yrs
2. Pregnant – teratogenic (e.g. DES)

CANCERS
Associated with ESTROGEN

1. ENDOMETRIAL CANCER
a. If EST alone – Inc risk 15 times
b. EST – Inc proliferation endometrium
   → hyperplastic endometrium
     premalignant – Inc risk of cancer
c. Risk is avoided completely by
   coadministering PROGESTIN
   (PROG Δ endometrium
     → secreting, can be shed)
d. Oral Contraceptives (EST/PROG)
   Have a lower risk of endometrium
   CA than those NOT taking OC

2. BREAST CANCER
   NO Inc risk with Oral Contraceptives

3. CERVICAL ADENOCARCINOMA
a. Inc risk if exposed while *in utero*
b. DES mother / daughter Inc risk
c. All exogenous EST – teratogenic
   NOT just DES

MORTALITY ASSOCIATED WITH OC

Regardless of smoking history, is
significantly lower than mortality
associated with child birth /
pregnancy

Smoke and age > 35 yrs
Mortality significantly Inc
Contraindicated

ESTROGENS	ESTRADIOL [327]	ESTRONE [328]	ESTRIOL [329]	SYNTHETIC STEROIDAL EST [330]
ADMINISTRATION	Oral – Micronized 1st pass effect	Oral – Micronized 1st pass effect	Oral – Micronized 1st pass effect	ETHINYL ESTRADIOL MESTRANOL QUINESTROL
	Most potent Major secretory product of the ovary Produced from testosterone	Comes from the liver	Produced from estradiol Most EST in this form	Oral Decreased 1st pass effect Only synthetic EST used in oral contraceptives (OC)
EFFECTS	Stimulation of 2° sex characteristics At puberty, stimulates release of HGH → growth spurt Closure of epiphyseal plate Development of the endometrial lining	Dec LH release, Dec androgens Dec bone reabsorption (PTH antagonist) Dec LDL's, Inc HDL's		OC contraindicated in: • Active liver disease • Tx of breast cancer

SYNTHETIC NONSTEROIDAL EST [331]

DIETHYLSTILBESTROL (DES)
CHLOROTRIANISENE
METHALLENESTRIL

Oral, NO 1st pass effect, good absorption
Much slower metabolism
Enters enterohepatic circulation (DES)

Exogenous ESTs can cause:
• Cervical adenocarcinoma
• Clear-cell carcinoma of the vagina (DES) in female offspring

CONJUGATED ESTROGENS

CONJUGATED ESTRADIOL
CONJUGATED ESTRONE
CONJUGATED ESTRIOL

Oral
Natural ESTs with sulfate group on the OH-
Decreased 1st pass effect

ESTROGENS	ESTRADIOL [327]	ESTRONE [328]
TREATMENT	Replacement Tx postmenopausal Osteoporosis Androgen-dependent tumors (Prostatic CA)	Oral contraceptives • Most common use Keeps LH, FSH, PROG, and EST levels low Inhibits ovulation • no LH surge
SIDE EFFECTS	MINOR 1. Nausea 2. Headaches 3. Postmenopausal bleeding 4. Alters serum proteins 5. Inc blood glucose Use more insulin if IDDM Contraindicated: pregnancy	MAJOR 1. Fluid retention – Stimulates angiotensin 2. Mild HT in 30% patients taking EST, by Inc aldoster Contraindicated: >40 yrs or >35 yrs smoker 3. Gallbladder disease – Causes bile to thicken, conc 4. Clotting disorders – Inc Factors II, VII, X & fibrinogen 2 – 3 x higher incidence stroke, NOT given to the elderly 5. Inc risk MI with risk factors: obesity, smoking, IDDM 6. Hyperplastic endometrium – premalignant Tx: use Progesterone → Secretory 7. Cancer – teratogenic

OTHER FEM STEROIDALS	PROGESTINS [332] PROGESTERONE	ORAL [333] CONTRACEPTIVES	TAMOXIFEN [334]	CLOMIPHENE [335]	RU - 486 [336]
ADMINISTRATION	Oral (OC) IM (oil depot)	Oral (E2 + P2)			
MECHANISM	Anti-Estrogen effect Large 1st pass effect	Inhibits ovulation Pseudopregnancy	Anti-Estrogen Effect	Anti-Estrogen effect	Anti-Progesterone effect
EFFECTS	Early intermed of steroids Promotes secretory endo Prevents implantation Contributes to lactation Progestin Properties: • Estrogenic & Antiestrog • Androgenic & Antiandro • Progestational	+EST to stop proliferative phase of endometrium Endometrium inappropriate for implantation Suppress synthesis of: EST, Prog, FL, FSH	Binds EST receptor at cellular level Displaces EST NO intrinsic action Binds both : Estrogen receptors Progesterone receptors	Binds EST receptor at the hypothalamus Dec (-) feedback → Inc GnRH → pituitary → Inc LH & FSH	Binds progesterone receptors PROG required for maintaining pregnancy
	OC Minipill if used alone Low Dose – Inhib implant High – Inhib Ovulation, EST DO NOT use in young females • Ovaries need long recovery time	**SIDE EFFECTS** • Hypertension • Fluid retention • Clotting disorder • Myocardial infarction • Breast CA(f)		**SIDE EFFECT** May cause a multiple gestational pregnancy (twins, triplets, . . .)	
TREATMENT	1. Endometriosis 2. Chronic anovulatory uterine bleeding 3. OC	Oral Contraceptives Contraindicated: Smokers > 35 yrs Pregnancy	Breast CA • EST-dependent tumor • 30 – 50% breast CA are EST or PROG (+)	Infertility	Abortion

OXYTOCIC	OXYTOCIN [337]	METHYLERGONOVINE ERGONOVINE [338]	PGE₂ [339]	PGF₂ₐ [340]
ADMINISTRATION	Endogenous IV	IM	Vaginal suppository	Suppository, Gel, Injection
DURATION	$T_{1/2} = 3$ min	$T_{1/2} = 2 - 3$ hrs	$T_{1/2} = 12 - 24$ hrs	Very potent Severe contractions
EFFECTS (Contract Uterus)	Milk let down, ejection Labor • Uterine contractions • Helps birth and expels placenta • Prevents postpartum hemorrhage by causing hemostasis • Rhythmic contractions NO Oxytocin receptors in early pregnancy ∴ No effect • NOT used for abortion	Longer $T_{1/2}$ Sustained contractions of the uterus can kill the neonate	Uterine effacement • Ripening the cervix for labor Cervix: cylinder → funnel High Concentration PGE₂ • Uterine contraction • NOT used	
SIDE EFFECTS	Ruptured uterus Hypotension (bolus injection) ADH properties – Dec urine volume Neonatal hyperbilirubinemia	Hypertension (IV) • Vasoconstriction	PGE₁ – used to maintain a patent ductus arteriosus	
TREATMENTS	1. Induce labor 2. Postpartum hemorrhage 3. Uterine atony • Uterus fails to contract, failure of labor contraction, hemorrhage, shock	Can induce labor, but NOT used for postpartum hemorrhage (atonia) if OXYTOCIN fails	Postpartum hemorrhage (from atonia), if both OXYTOCIN and ERGONOVINE fail	Induce abortions (usually 2nd trimester) Postpartum hemorrhage (from atonia), if all other drugs listed fail

TOCOLYTICS	MAGNESIUM SULFATE [341]	RITODRINE [342]	TERBUTALINE [343]	ETHANOL [344]
ADMINISTRATION	IV	IV Oral	NOT FDA Approved	Oral NO longer used
MECHANISM (Relax uterus)	Antagonizes Ca^{++} Arrests labor	β_2 agonist Stimulates cAMP synthesis in the uterine myometrial cells Stimulates Ca^{++} and Mg^{++} – dependent ATPase	β_2 agonist Stimulates cAMP synthesis Stimulates Ca^{++} and Mg^{++} – ATPase	
EFFECTS	Monitor for signs of toxicity			
SIDE EFFECTS	Mg^{++} Toxicity • 1st sign – loss of reflexes • Cessation of breathing • Cardiac arrest Rx: Ca gluconate – infuse large amounts quickly, Ca^{++} will displace Mg^{++}	Pulmonary edema • Must restrict fluid intake	Pulmonary edema	
TREATMENT	Inhibits contraction of uterus Prevents premature labor Counteracts oxytocic drugs	Inhibits contraction of uterus Prevents premature labor Counteracts oxytocic drugs	Inhibits contraction of uterus Prevents premature labor Counteracts oxytocic drugs	Inhibits contraction Prevents premature labor Counteracts oxytocic drugs

	ORAL HYPOGLYCEMIC	GLYBURIDE GLIPIZIDE [346]
	DURATION	Onset = 1 – 2 hr $T_{1/2}$ = 1 – 2 days
	DRUG INTERACTIONS	2nd generation 1° action: Inc number of receptors More potent NOT highly protein-bound GLYBURIDE: 200 x TOLB Excreted: 50% bile, 50% urine Diuretic GLIPIZIDE: 100 x TOLB Excreted: urine Food delays absorption
	SIDE EFFECTS	Fewer side effects NO alcohol flushing
	TREATMENT	

PHENFORMIN

Reduces blood glucose

A biguinide anti-IDDM

NOT a sulfonylurea
 • Inc lactic acid
 • Inc ability of glucose to go into cells

Use:
1. Hyperglycemia
2. Weight reduction

COMMON SULFONAMIDES

1. Stim insulin release from β cells
2. Inhibit glucose release from glycogen stores in the liver
3. Inc number and/or sensitivity of insulin receptors
4. Most effective in new diabetics (lower doses)
5. Must have 25% of islets functioning
6. Do NOT work if NO pancreas, NO β cells, or IDDM

TOLBUTAMIDE (ORINASE®) [347]	ACETOHEXAMIDE (DYMELOR®) [348]	TOLAZAMIDE (TOLINASE®) [349]	CHLORPROPAMIDE (DIABINESE®) [350]
Onset = 1 hr $T_{1/2}$ = 9 ± 3 hr	Onset = 3 – 4 hr $T_{1/2}$ = 18 ± 6 hr	Onset = 4 – 6 hr $T_{1/2}$ = 18 ± 6 hr	Onset = 3 – 4 hr $T_{1/2}$ = 36 ± 3 hr
Binds plasma proteins • Albumin • Watch for drug Interaction Chronic use • Dec effectiveness	Plasma protein pound Metabolized to an active intermediate • Extends duration Uricosuric • Inc uric acid excret • May help gout Diuretic	Plasma protein bound Diuretic	Plasma protein bound Antidiuretic action • Epilepsy • CHF • Inc ADH – Inc P°
Any Drug that displaces oral hypoglycemics from protein : causes Dec blood sugar: • PHENYTOIN (antiinflammatory) • CLOFIBRATE (antilipemic)	Drugs that Inc blood sugar require Inc dose oral hypoglycemic: • CORTICOSTEROIDS • ESTROGENS • ORAL CONTRACEPTIVES		Interactions with O.T.C. drugs potentiate hypoglycemia Anything with alcohol (e.g. cough syrup) causes flushing

1. Hypoglycemia
  • Misuse and inappropriate diet
2. Skin reaction photosensitivity
3. Abnormal liver cholestatic jaundice, elevated liver enzymes
4. Transient leukopenia thrombocytopenia
 	
NOT teratogenic, but do NOT use if pregnant
Pregnant: D.O.C. is insulin
 	
CONTRAINDICATED
  1. Pregnancy
  2. Pancreatectomy
  3. IDDM
  4. Phenylbutazone
			1. Hypoglycemia Misuse and inappropriate diet
			2. Skin Reaction Photosensitivity
			3. Abnormal liver Cholestatic jaundice Elevated liver enzymes
			4. Transient leukopenia Thrombocytopenia
			5. Water Retention complicates CHF and epilepsy
			6. Because of long duration, cumulative effects (i.e. hypoglycemic shock)
			7. Disulfiram reaction

NIDDM	NIDDM
	Gout
		NIDDM
		Hypertension
			CONTRAINDICATED
			  1. CHF
			  2. Epilepsy
			  3. Alcohol
			  4. Pregnancy
			  5. Pancreatectomy
			  6. IDDM
			  7. Phenylbutazone

HYPOTHYROID	THYROID USP [351]	LEVOTHYROXINE [352]	LIOTHYRONINE [353]	LIOTRIX [354]
TYPE	Natural – Animal thyroid T_3 and T_4 • Oral • 100% absorption	Synthroid® Synthetic T_4 Oral • 40 – 70% absorption	Cytomel® Synthetic T_3 Oral • 100% absorption	Combination of LEVOTHYROXINE and LIOTHYRONINE Oral
DURATION	Onset: 24 hrs $T_{1/2}$ = 4 – 5 days Potency: 1/25 – 1/35	Onset: 2 days $T_{1/2}$ = 9 days Potency: 1 (= thyroxine)	Onset: 12 –18 hrs $T_{1/2}$ = 2 days Potency = 3 – 8 x	
	Dose: 120 mg – 180 mg (others in µg) • Very weak drug	Effective dose: 200 – 300 µg/day T_4 peripheral conversion to T_3	Fast acting Inc metabolism rate 40 Units / 24 hr	NO Advantage
USE	Use: replacement Tx Hypothyroidism	D.O.C.: replacement Tx Hypothyroidism	Use: drug induced hypothyroidism	
TOXICITY	Side effects: • Thyrotoxicosis • Tachycardia • Inc BP° • Nervousness			

Iodination of tyrosine is most important step

THYROID OVERDOSE
Thyrotoxicosis symptoms (Inc BP°, angina, tachycardia, palpitations, nervous, weight loss, insomnia, sweating)

CONTRAINDICATED
Extreme caution with cardiovascular disease. Discontinue if pain occurs

---

HYPOFUNCTION

1. Cretinism – child
2. Myxedema
3. Hashimoto's disease – autoimmune
4. Simple goiter

SYMPTOMS
Cold intolerance, paresthesia, lethargy, loss of libido, dry skin, dec growth & maturity (child), retardation

---

HYPERFUNCTION (thyrotoxicosis)

1. Grave's Disease
2. Goiter

SYMPTOMS
Tachycardia, sweat, tremble, eyelids droop, clubbed fingers

HYPERTHYROID	K PERCHLORATE [355] Na THIOCYANATE	METHIMAZOLE (METH) [356] PROPYLTHIOURACIL (PTU)	RADIOACTIVE [357] IODINE	LUGOL'S SOLUTION [358]
	IONIC INHIBITORS Inhibit trapping mechanism Iodine can't be taken up No longer used	**THIOAMIDES** Interferes with iodination of tyrosyl 1. Inhibits peroxidase system, blocks the conversion of iodide to active compound 2. Inhibit coupling • Block coupling of MIT + DIT → TIT DIT + DIT → Thyroxine 3. Blocks the peripheral conversion of $T_4 → T_3$ • PTU only, (NOT METHIMAZOLE) These drugs do NOT block the release of T_3 and T_4 METH is 10 x more potent than PTU Remission: after a year, withdraw – get a relapse Cured: NO relapse after 2 – 3 yr when withdraw drug	Emits β and γ rays $T_{1/2}$ = 8 days Dose dependent ^{131}I is preferentially taken up by thyroid, acts on colloid 70% respond to one dose Too Little → NO effect Too Much → Destroys gland → hypothyroidism	10% KI Antagonizes TSH 1. Blocks release of T_3 and T_4 2. Inhibits iodide pump by affecting TSH **USE** Presurgically • 10 days PreOp • Reduces size and vascularity of goiter
	PROPRANOLOL [359] β blocker Relieves palpitation, nervousness, anxiety, tachycardia Inhibits conversion of $T_4 → T_3$ peripherally Reduces symptoms of hyperthyroidism Does NOT become euthyroid	**SIDE EFFECTS** Skin rash, nausea, vomiting (oral), agranulocytosis, drug fever OD – First sign of hypothyroidism reduce dose/ discontinue **CONTRAINDICATED** Pregnancy • Neonatal goiter/hypothyroidism **PTU SIDE EFFECT** Inc size and vascularity of the thyroid gland	**ADVANTAGES** 1. NO surgery, NO trauma 2. Good for elderly and cardiac patients 3. Patients who have relapsed **CONTRAINDICATED** 1. Pregnancy 2. Children • Cretinism • Myxedema **SIDE EFFECT** Hypothyroidism	**SURGICAL ABLATION** 80 – 90% cured by removing ⅞ of the thyroid **COMPLICATIONS** • 3% Mortality • 4 – 30% Hypothyroidism • Hypoparathyroid (rare) • 4% Vocal cord paralysis • Cosmetic disfigurement Only use if all other methods fail

PARATHYROID REGULATION	PARATHYROID HORMONE [361]	HYPERPARATHYROID [362]
CAUSES	Maintain ECF Ca^{++} • Inc plasma Ca^{++} level	85% Single adenoma 15% Hyperplasia
EFFECTS **MECHANISM**	1. Inc $Ca^{++}/PO_4^{=}$ reabsorption from bone → mobilizes bone Ca^{++} 2. Inc Ca^{++} reabsorption from kidney 3. Inc $PO_4^{=}$ excretion 4. Inc Ca^{++} absorption from GI tract 5. Inc Vit D_3 synthesis Inc osteoclast metabolism • Inc acid → demineralize • 2° Inc of osteoblasts • Inc bone turnover rate Ca^{++} level regulates the synthesis, growth, secretion of the parathyroid to maintain normal Ca^{++} level of 4.5 – 5.3 meq/l. $Ca^{++} < 3 – 4$ meq → Inc PTH $Ca^{++} > 6$ meq/l → Dec PTH PTH: Inc Ca^{++}, Dec $PO_4^{=}$ Vit D → 1,25 Di(OH) D • Inc Ca^{++}, Inc $PO_4^{=}$	Ca^{++} level > 7 meq/l SIGNS 1. GI upset, abdominal pain, peptic ulcers 2. Renal calculi stones, pain 3. CNS: headaches, depression, psychiatric manifestations 4. Cardiac arrhythmia
TOXICITY	SIDE EFFECTS GI upset, abdominal pain, renal calculi, renal damage, CNS disturbances	SIDE EFFECTS Surgery – can result in hypoparathyroidism Rx: Vit D + Ca^{++}
USES	USES Synthetic PTH Diagnostic only DDx: Pseudohypoparathyroidism NOT predictable for Tx	TX 1. Surgery – Choice Tx • Remove ⅓ gland • Remove adenoma 2. Drugs to lower [Ca^{++}] a. Diuretics • FUROSEMIDE • ETHACRYNIC ACID • Inc Ca^{++} excretion b. MITHRAMYCIN • Inhibits osteoclasts c. GLUCOCORTICOIDS • Antagonize Vit D • Dec Ca^{++} absorption d. CALCITONIN • Inhibits bone resorption

---

CALCIUM IONS

Important for:
• Neuromuscular function
• Cardiac function
• Coagulation
• Bone structure

Increased requirements for:
• Children
• Pregnant women
• Post-menopausal females

Ionized, unbound Ca^{++} is active

HYPOPARATHYROID [363]	VITAMIN D [364]	CALCITONIN [365]

1. Surgery/trauma
2. Hypofunction
3. Genetic defect
   Pseudohypoparathyroidism
	Necessary for
	  Ca^{++} absorption
		Antagonist of PTH

Pseudohypoparathyroidism
 	
target organs do NOT
  respond
 	
SYMPTOMS
• Paraesthesia
• Short stature
• Mental retardation
• Laryngospasm
• Convulsions
• Tachycardia
• Hair loss
• Brittle nails
• Cataracts
• Psychosis
 	
<div style="border:1px solid">Give Ca^{++} salts slowly
to avoid arrhythmia</div>
	Synthesized by skin, liver
	  and kidney together
	Oral administration
	
	Vit D deficiency
	• Inc PTH
	• Loss of bone
	Child: rickets
	• Fail to mineralize
	Adult: osteomalacia
	• Dec bone density
	INTERACTIONS
	1. Anticonvulsants
	   PHENYTOIN
	   PHENOBARBITAL
	   • Inc metab Vit D
	   • Dec Vit D activity
	2. Glucocorticoids
	  • Antagonize Vit D
	SIDE EFFECTS
	Hypervitaminosis D
	1. Hypercalcemia
	  • Weakness, fatigue
	2. Calcification of
	  soft tissues
	CONTRAINDICATED
	• Anticonvulsants
		Secreted by C cells
		  Parafollicular thyroid
		
		1. Dec Plasma Ca^{++}
		2. Directly inhibits bone
		  resorption
		  • Inhibits osteoclasts
		3. Stim bone synthesis
		  • Stim osteoblasts
		4. Inhibits renal
		  excretion of Ca^{++}
		
		SIDE EFFECTS
		1. GI upset: nausea,
		  vomiting, diarrhea
		2. Inflammation at
		  injection Site

TX
1. <u>VIT D</u> – Oral
• Bile necessary for Vit D absorp
• Dihydrotachysterol
  Vit D analog
  rapid mobilization of bone salts
• Calcitriol – Vit D_3
 	
2. <u>CALCIUM SALTS</u>
• Ca salt + Vit D – for Tx of
  hypocalcemia tetany
• Ca gluconate (D.O.C.) – best
  against tetany, does NOT
  irritate at IV site
• Ca chloride (IV) – irritates at IV
  site
• Synthetic PTH – DDx Pseudo-
  hypoparathyroidism
	**DIHYDRO-
	TACHYSTEROL [366]**
	
	Vit D analog
	Greater effect on bones
	
	USES / TX:
	1. Rickets
	2. Osteomalacia
	3. Hypoparathyroidism
	4. Vit D deficiency
		USES / TX:
		1. Hyperparathyroidism
		  • Vit D intoxication
		2. Paget's Disease
		  • Blocks bone
		  resorption and Dec
		  pain
		
		Long Term Tx is well
		tolerated
		
		May develop resistance

6 ANTIBIOTICS

URINARY TRACT INFECTIONS [222]	METHENAMINE [223]	NALIDIXIC ACID [224]
CYSTITIS One of the most common infections • Moist, dark, low 0_2 tension *E. coli* #1 agent • Use SULFA drug or combination of SULFONAMIDE & TRIMETHOPRIM Recurrent infections: 1. Diabetics 2. Anomaly 3. Protected site (Prostate)	Bacteriocidal Given systemically Acts 1° on urinary tract Infections Spectrum: Lower UT, *E. coli* *Proteus* (Non indole +) (Indol + – Inc pH) FORMALDEHYDE • Precipitates proteins • Embalming METHENAMINE • Breaks down to 4 NH_4 + 6 FORMALDEHYDES ORAL NO Signif Decomp in GI tract Decomposition is pH dependent Intact in the Blood, but decomposes in Lower UT – acidic Slow breakdown = 3 hr MECHANISM FORMALD denatures proteins (works on spores and bacteria) Must maintain acid pH urine: • Mandelate • Hippuric acid • Ascorbic acid SIDE EFFECTS • Ammonia release • Hematuria • Proteinuria CONTRAINDICATED WITH • Liver disease • Renal disease (crystalluria) • Dehydration (crystalluria) • Can give METHENAMINE with renal disease, but do NOT also give organic acid (Mandelate) – crystalluria – bicarbonate pH DRUG INTERACTION • Do NOT use with any SULFA drugs (Sulfanilamide) • Inactivates and insolubilizes (Crystalluria) 1° USE Chronic suppressive Tx of recurrent UTI	Bacteriocidal $T_{1/2}$ = 8 hr 97% albumen bound (∴ little or NO systemic effect) Topoisomerase inhibitor (Gyrase) • Replication • Repair • Recombination • Transposition (Opens supercoil 4° structural Δ) Absorbed well, T = 8 hr SPECTRUM: ORAL • *E. coli* • *Proteus* • *Klebsiella* NOT *Pseudomonas* (resistant) NOT systemically effective (*Proteus*) Plasma protein bound METABOLISM (20%) • Hydroxylated to OXYNALIDIX (Cyto P_{450}) • Inc activity • Conjugated (80%) glucuronic acid • Inactive EXCRETION • Excreted highly in the kidney OXYNALIDIX is active • Does NOT penetrate the prostate gland. • Filtered & secreted, be careful in renal insufficiency SIDE EFFECTS 1. GI upset 2. CNS: headache, vertigo, ataxia, convulsions at high doses 3. Skin: allergy, photosensitive CONTRAINDICATIONS • Pregnancy • Nursing women • Children (Inc intracranial P°) DRUG INTERACTION • NITROFURANTOIN – cancel each other out

FLUOROQUINOLONES [225]		NITROFURANTOIN [226]	PHENAZOPYRIDINE [227]
NORFLOXACIN	**CIPROFLOXACIN**		

NORFLOXACIN	CIPROFLOXACIN	NITROFURANTOIN	PHENAZOPYRIDINE
1° for urinary tract infection Oral 20 – 40% absorbed Erratic Filtered and secreted rapidly into urine	USE UTIs, bone, respiratory, skin Oral better absorbed (Unique – oral for systemic infection Fluoride atom – Dec resistance	Bacteriocidal Bacteriostatic (depends on conc) Good for *E. coli* and Gram (+) & (-) NOT *Pseudomonas, Klebsiella, Proteus, Enterobacter*	NOT antiseptic Urinary tract analgesia (relieves pain) • Dec dysuria • Dec burning • Dec urgency

Inhibit Gram (+) & Gram (-) aerobes
  (Broad spectrum antibiotic)
USE against penicillinase-producing
    organisms
• *Pseudomonas* · few resistant strains
    · Chromosomal Δ · enzyme
• METHICILLIN-resistant Staphylococci
• *Legionnaire's* pneumonia
• *Enterobacter*
• *Klebsiella*
• *Shigella* – CIPROFLOXACIN
NOT ANAEROBES – resistant

MECHANISM
Interferes with energy producing e⁻ transfer in pyruvate metabolism

METABOLISM
Completely absorbed
• Excreted mostly unchanged – urine
• Rapid excretion
• $T_{1/2}$ = 20 – 60 min
• Cleaved by reduction reaction in bacteria
• Product interferes with DNA synthesis
If impaired renal function → adjust dose / time

SIDE EFFECTS
1. Red urine
2. GI upset
3. Methemoglobinemia

SIDE EFFECTS
1. GI upset
2. CNS effects – rare
3. Arthropathy – destroy cartilage in weight-bearing joints

CONTRAINDICATED
        • Pregnancy
        • Nursing Women
        • Children

CIPROFLOXACIN
  Inhibits metabolism
  of THEOPHYLLINE
  (in Asthma Tx)

SIDE EFFECTS
1. GI upset
2. Tx: milk or macrocrystalline
3. Leukopenia, granulocytopenia
4. Elderly: allergic pneumonia, Interstitial fibrosis
5. NO_2 containing
6. Hemolytic anemia G-6-P DH deficiency (X linked)
7. Neuro Effects:
a. IRREVERSIBLE
    • Peripheral polyneuropathy (sensory & balance)
    • Paresthesia
    • Loss of balance
    Demyelination, axon loss (withdraw drug)
b. REVERSIBLE
    • Headache
    • Vertigo
    • Nystagmus
May Inhibit e⁻ TS of pyruvate
Resistance – rare
    • Dec recurring infection
Brown urine
Rapidly excreted

SULFONAMIDES[228]

BACTERIOSTATIC

USES:
1. UTIs – SULFISOXAZOLE
2. Pulmonary Infection due to *Nocardia*
3. Trachoma (Conjunctivitis)
4. Toxoplasmosis • PYRIMETHAMINE
   (DHF Reductase Inhibitor)
5. *Pneumocystis carinii* • TRIMETHOPRIM
   • AIDS patients
6. *Plasmodium* • Chloroquine-resistant *P. falc*
   • use PYRIMETHAMINE
7. *Chlamydia* • 1° in UTI
8. Penicillin-sensitive patients
9. Colitis • SULFASALAZINE (Azulfidine®)
10. Meningococcal meningitis
11. *Salmonella typhosa* • now resistant to others

PROPHYLAXIS
1. Maxillo facial trauma (*Rhinorrhea, Otorrhea*)
2. Burns, prevent *Pseudomonas* (Sulfamylon)
3. Rheumatic fever

DEVELOPMENT
AZO DYES (Prontosil®) Prodrug becomes reduced
to SULFANILAMIDE (active) Bacteriostatic
Broad Spectrum (Gram(+) and Gram(-))

STRUCTURAL REQUIREMENTS
1. Benzene derivative
2. Requires free amino group – para (N^4)
3. NO substitutions on the ring
4. Substitution permitted on the N^1
   Substitutions alter: • Physiologic properties (pKa)
   • Pharmacokinetics (absorb, metab) • Solubility
   in water • It will NOT Δ spectrum of activity

MECHANISM
A. Reaction in bacteria:
1. Pteridine + PABA → dihydropteroic acid
   • *SULFAS block here   (DHP A)
   • Pteroic acid synthetase
*Selective against bacteria (mammals do not make it)
B. Bacteria and Mammals
2. DHP Acid → dihydrofolic acid (DHF)
3. DHF (or FAH_2) → tetrahydrofolate
   (THF or FAH_4)
   – TRIMETHOPRIM works here – DHF reductase
4. Inhibits formation of: thymidine → DNA
   Purines → RNA, DNA
   Methionine, glycine, f -Met tRNA → proteins
Bacteriostatic – inhibits growth
 If in necrotic area, cell products released can be
 used to replace those SULF blocks – decrease
 effectiveness of SULFs – drain abscess first

PHARMACOKINETICS
• Well absorbed in GI, plasma
  protein-bound
• Used systemically
• Into body fluids: synovial
  CNS, UT, placenta, milk
• Metab to inactive compounds
  (liver)
•Para-Amino → NAc derivative
  Less soluble → crystalluria

TOXICITY: CRYSTALLURIA
NOT very H_2O Soluble because:
• Weak acids (anion) pKa ~ 10
• If urine pH ~ 7
   $$10 = 7 + \log [P]/[NP]$$
   $$= 1000 [P] : 1 [NP]$$
P = protonated,
   crystallizes – kidney problems
NP = nonP, charged – preferred

SULFISOXAZOLE pKa = 7
1 P : 1 NP H_2O Soluble
New drugs: Lower pKa, more soluble,
                compet inhibit PABA

TO AVOID CRYSTALLURIA
1. New drugs have lower pKa
2. Good body hydration
3. Alkalinize the urine – Ion trap 4.
*TRIPLE SULFAs
5. Bound to plasma proteins
   Dec pKa → Inc %PPB

SIDE EFFECTS OF PLASMA PROTEIN
BINDING
1. Bilirubin competitively displaced
   • Jaundice (adult)
   • Kernicterus (neonatal brain)
   Destroys neurons,
   Basal ganglia, dyskinesia
2. Other drugs displaced
• Oral Anticoagulants
• Methotrexate

OTHER TOXICITY
1. Allergy • dermal/topical (3 – 10%)
2. Oral – Stevens-Johnson syndrome, exfoliative dermatitis – rash
3. G-6-P DH deficiency – hemolytic
   anemia

CONTRAINDICATED
1. Pregnancy
2. Infants
3. Impaired liver or kidney
   function (alcoholic)
4. Prior history of sulfanil allergy
5. Do NOT use with METHENAMINE

DRUGS

SULFISOXAZOLE – Inc urine solubility (UTIs)
SULFAMETHOXAZOLE – Use with TRIMETHOPRIM
  Synergistic effect (UTI)
  Combination is better than
    alone, broader spectrum   **SMZ**
  20 Sulfamethoxazole: **MIC**
    1 Trimethoprim
  • Inc efficacy   **TMP MIC**
  • Dec resistance development

TRIMETHOPRIM:
• Inhibits DHF reductase (eukaryotes, too) but bacterial enzyme has a greater affinity
• Well absorbed, gets into PROSTATE
• Uses: *UTI, *P. carinii*, toxoplasma malaria, *Shigella*

CONCENTRATION 50% INHIBITION (DHF Reductase)

Drug	Human	*E.coli*	*P. berghei*
TRIMETHOPRIM	300,000	5	70
PYRIMETHAMINE	1,800	2,500	0.5

PYRIMETHAMINE – Antimalarial activity
TOXICITY same as SULFANILAMIDE

CONTRAINDICATED Folic acid deficiency
• Pregnancy
• Malnourishment } Causes megaloblastic anemia
• Alcoholics   Give folic acid
                (bacteria can't use, except *Enterococci*)

SULFACETAMIDE (topical) trachoma – eye, pH = 7.4 in solution
SILVER SULFADIAZINE (topical) for burns
MAFENIDE (topical), more potent, burns – can inhibit metabolic acidosis

SULFASALAZINE – Inflammatory bowel disease – a salicylate product
USE
  1. Urinary tract infections – SULFISOXAZOLE
  2. Pulmonary infection due to *Nocardia*
  3. Trachoma (conjunctivitis)
  4. Toxoplasmosis – PYRIMETHAMINE (DHF reductase inhibitor)
  5. *Pneumocystis carinii* – TRIMETHOPRIM
  6. *Plasmodium* – Chloroquine-resistant *P. falciparum* – use PYRIMETHAMINE
  7. *Chlamydia* – 1 ° in urinary tract infection

Susceptible organisms must synthesize and utilize their own folic acid

SULFONAMIDES
1. High solubility, low toxicity: SULFACETAMIDE, SULFISOXAZOLE
2. Remain largely unabsorbed, Δ bacterial flora: SUCCINYL & SULFAMETHIZOLE
3. Rapidly absorbed, slowly excreted: SULFADIMETHOXINE,
    SULFAMETHOXYPYRIDAZINE
4. Combinations with antibiotics and TRIMETHOPRIM

PENICILLINS [229]
(in General)

All have a 4 membered, β - lactam ring
- Essential for activity
- Fused to a 5 membered thiazolidine ring
- All have sulfur, carboxyl or acidic groups

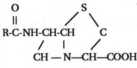

6-aminopenicillanic acid

- R group determines stability to enzyme or acid hydrolysis and affects the antibacterial spectrum
- Na⁺ or K⁺ salts of PEN are soluble
- Procaine or Benzathine esters are insoluble – depot preparations

ADMINISTRATION
Determined by:
- Stability in gastric acid
- Severity of infection

Oral: NOT with meals, either 30 – 60 min before, or 2 hours after (especially with PEN G). Higher gastric pH (less acid) in children/elderly → Inc absorption. Lower gastric pH (Inc acid) of Zollinger-Ellison syndrome → Dec absorption.

USEFUL
1. Diabetics with infections
2. Chronic liver disease
3. Cancer chemotherapy
4. AIDS

MECHANISM OF ACTION
- Inhibits cell wall (peptidoglycan) synthesis by interfering with transpeptidation
- Gram (-) NOT very effective. Penicillinase between cytoplasmic membrane and peptidoglycan
- Gram (+) NO cell wall. Penicillinase elaborated into the medium
- Problem with mixed infections
- Antibiotic gets into cytoplasm – UDP-Mur-NAc pentapeptide accumulators
- All bacteriocidal in growing cells only
- Interfere with cell wall synthesis by inhibiting the transpeptidation step.
- PBPs (Penicillin Binding Proteins) are responsible for cell wall synthesis. Penicillin's binding changes morphology or causes lysis.

MECHANISM OF RESISTANCE
1. NO PG in the cell wall
2. β-lactamase plasmid or chromosome
3. NOT taken up by the bacteria
4. Alters the PBP (e.g. MRSA)
- Methicillin resistant Staphylococci
- Use:

     VANCOMYCIN,
     RIFAMPIN,
     CIPROFLOXACIN

IRREVERSIBLE INHIBITORS OF B-LACTAMASE
1. CLAVULANIC ACID
2. SULBACTAM
- Formulated with Amoxicillin, Ticarcillin and Ampicillin
- Changes spectrum

DICLOXACILLIN
- Best Absorbed
- May lead to osteomyelitis

DISTRIBUTION
- Binds albumin
- Penetrates all body fluids
- Inc penetrance when inflamed
- CNS when inflamed meninges
- All cross placenta, but are safe
- Into bones
- NOT prostate
- Does NOT displace other drugs
- NO interaction

BILIARY TRACT INFECTION
(*E. coli*)
AMPICILLIN
IMIPENEM,
AZTREONAM

IV or IM (NOT Oral)
METHICILLIN, CARBENICILLIN, IMIPENEM, AZTREONAM,

All antipseudomonal penicillins:
CARBENICILLIN, TICARCILLIN, PIPERACILLIN

PENICILLINS [229]
(in General)

B-LACTAM ANTIBIOTICS
- Act synergistically with aminoglycosides
- Never put into same IV bottle, they will inactivate each other

METABOLISM
- Insignificant in the host
- IMIPENEM is metab in proximal renal tubule by dehydropeptidase (nephrotoxic)
- CILASTATIN will inhibit enzyme

EXCRETION
1. 1° renal route
- Organic acid secretion system
- Glomerular filtration PROBENECID
- Dec secretion of PENs and CARBAPENAMs
- Inc $T_{1/2}$
2. Hepatobiliary route
  *NAFCILLIN – excreted AMPICILLIN, PIPERACILLIN, AZTREONAM recirculation

TOXICITY
1. Hypersensitivity reactions
   Rash ↔ Anaphylaxis
   PEN G → Benzylpenicillinic acid + lysine → hapten
2. AMPICILLIN
   - maculopapular rash
   - pathognomonic for mononucleosis
3. Diarrhea
   - Antibiotic induced colitis
     C. difficile or Inc Staph → pseudomembranous colitis – AUGMENTIN®
4. Acute interstitial nephritis
   - High dose METHICILLIN
5. Induce seizures by irritating neuro
   - Interferes with GABA – PEN G and IMIPENEM/CILASTATIN. Contraindicated: epileptics
6. Platelet dysfunction – Dec agglutination
   - Antipseudomonal PENs and to a degree with PEN G
   - Potentiates anticoagulants and is important in uremic patients
7. Eosinophilia, leukopenia
   - ACYL UREDO PENICILLINS
8. False positives
   - Urinary glucose oxidase test (AUGMENTIN®)
9. Other toxicities NOT due to PEN, but due to the nature of the salts – Cardiotoxicity
10. Hypokalemia – CARBENICILLIN

PENICILLINASE

Gram (-) : Between cytoplasmic membrane & peptidoglycan

Gram (+) : Elaborated into the medium

PENICILLINS	BENZYL PENICILLINS [230]	EXTENDED SPECTRUM [231]

DRUGS	PENICILLIN G
	PENICILLIN V
	
	ORAL
	• Acid stable
	• PENase sensitive
		AMPICILLIN
		AMOXICILLIN
		  (better absorb)
		AUGMENTIN®
		  (AMOX+ Clav)
		AMP + Sulbact

STABILITY	PENICILLIN G
	D.O.C.: Gram (-) cocci
	Staph without PENase
	  Cellulitis, osteomyelitis,
	  Meningococcal meningitis,
	  Clostridium perfringens,
	  Clostridium tetani, Syphilis,
	  Lyme disease, pneumonitis
		ORAL
		• Acid stable
		• PENase stable
		  AMOX + Clavulanate
		  AMP + Sulbactam

ANTIBACTERIAL SPECTRUM	Gm (+) and (-)
	  Spirochaete, anaerobes
	Enter CNS when inflamed
	
	PENICILLIN V
	• like PEN G
	• NOT as potent
	• Better absorbed
	  Upper respiratory tract
	  infection
	NOT Effective:
	  E. coli, Proteus, Pseudomonas,
	  H. influenzae
	
	PROCAINE PEN G
	BENZATHINE PEN
	• I.M. PEN G derivative
	• Absorbed slowly
	• Low blood concentration
	• Long duration
	PROC PEN G – gonorrhea
	BENZ PEN G – prophylaxis,
	  Rheumatic fever, heart
	  disease, syphilis
		Gram (-) rods
		Non typhoid *Salmonella*
		Same as PEN G
		Wider range
		(NOT as potent)
		Gram(-): *E. coli, H. influenzae,*
		  Shigella, Salmonella
		
		Pediatric meningitis
		  D.O.C.: 3rd generation
		  Cephalosporins
		Listeria
		Adult meningitis
		  D.O.C.: Ampicillin
		Salmonella /Shigella
		  COTRIMOXAZOLE
		
		AUGMENTIN®
		1. Bite wounds
		2. *Bacteroides*
		3. *H. influenzae* (upper
		  respiratory tract infection)
		4. PENase production
		5. *Proteus*
		6. *Listeria*

SIDE EFFECTS
 	
TOXICITY
	PENICILLIN G:
	1. Irritates neuronal tissue
	  • Seizure (inhibits GABA)
	2. Platelet dysfunction
	3. Cardiac arrest w/ salt forms
	  • Na^+: expands ECF,
	    Inc cardiac work
	  • K^+: arrhythmia
	4. Allergic reaction
	  • Tx with EPI, 0.3 – 0.5 ml,
	    1: 1000 solution
		If well absorbed,
		  Less diarrhea (AMOXICIL)
		Tx of lower GI
		Salmonella /Shigella infections
		want poor absorption
		(AMPICLLIN)
		
		SIDE EFFECTS:
		1. Diarrhea • AUGMENTIN
		  • Clavulanic acid
		2. False + oral glucose
		  tolerance test
		3. Maculopapular rash
		  (AMPICILLIN)

ANTISTAPH PENICILLINS [232]	ANTIPSEUDOMONAL [233]	CARBAPENEMS [234]	MONOBACTAMS [235]
METHICILLIN (IV Administer) DICLOXACILLIN CLOXACILLIN OXACILLIN NAFCILLIN	CARBENICILLIN CARBENICILLIN INDANYL TICARCILLIN - TIMENTIN® (TICAR + Clav Acid) PIPERACILLIN (Piperazine Penicillin) AZLOCILLIN (Ureido P) MEZLOCILLIN (Ureido P)	IMIPENEM PRIMAXIN® (IMIPENEM + CILASTATIN)	AZTREONAM
ORAL (except METH, IV) • Acid stable • PENase stable METH is NOT acid stable	IV • Acid labile (except CARBENICILLIN, which is acid stable) • PENase sensitive (except TIC + Clav A)	IV • Acid labile • PENase stable	IV • Acid labile • PENase stable
Gram (+) and (-) *H. influenzae* • Resists development PENase producing *Staph. aureus* Problem: (MRSA) METHICILLIN Resistant strains- alter Pen binding protein VANCOMYCIN Sensitive DICLOXACILLIN • Best absorbed • Osteomyelitis NAFCILLIN • Bile excreted	1° *Pseudomonas* 2° *Enterobacter* Gram(-) • *Klebsiella* - resistant chromo/constitutive • *E. coli* Usually used in combination with aminoglycosides PIPERACILLIN • Most potent • Dec Na⁺ load UREIDOPENICILLIN (AZLO & MEZLOCILLIN) • Acyl side chain • Δ spectrum (PEN G)	Broadest spectrum Gram (+) and (-) D.O.C.: • Actinetobacter • Anaerobes • Some *Pseudomonas* Treat fever of unknown origin NOT for: • *Pseudomonas multiformans* • *Pseudomonas cepacia* IMEPENEM • Metab by DHP nephrotoxic CILASTATIN • Inhibits DHP • Dec toxicity	Active against • Gram (-) aerobes NOT effective against: • Gram (+) anaerobes
METHICILLIN • Acute interstitial nephritis	SIDE EFFECTS 1. Platelet dysfunction 2. Eosinophilia 3. Leukopenia 4. Hypokalemia	SIDE EFFECT Seizure	

$$Gram (+) and (-)$$

GENERAL RULE

Acid Stable: ORAL

Acid Labile: IV, IM, IT

DRUGS EFFECTIVE AGAINST ANAEROBES

1. PENICILLIN G
2. CLINDAMYCIN
3. CEFOXITIN
4. METRONIDAZOLE
5. IMIPENEM

CEPHALOSPORINS [236]	1ST GENERATION	2ND GENERATION	3RD GENERATION
DRUGS	CEPHALOTHIN (IV) CEFAZOLIN (IV), (osteomyelitis) CEPHAPIRIN (IV) CEPHALEXIN (oral) CEPHRADINE (oral) CEFADROXIL (oral)	CEFAMANDOLE (bile) CEFOXITIN = CEPHAMYCIN CEFOTETAN CEFONICID (Inc $T_{1/2}$) CEFUROXIME (oral or IV), (CSF) CEFACLOR (oral)	CEFOTAXIME (CSF infection) MOXALACTAM (O instead of S) CEFOPERAZONE (bile) CEFTIZOXIME (osteomyelitis) CEFTRIAXONE (bile, CSF inf, Inc T) CEFTAZIDIME CEFIXIME (oral)

SPECTRUM OF ACTIVITY	Like PENICILLIN G – AMPICILLIN
	• a PEN substitute
	
	Active Against Gram (-) rods
	• *Proteus*
	• *E. coli* } "PEcK"
	• *Klebsiella*
	
	Active Against Gram (+)
	Strep. viridans
	Pneumococci
	Group A hemolytic *Strep*
	S. aureus
	
	NOT inactivated by PENase (*Staph*)
	
	Oral or IV
	IM – painful
	IT – NEVER inject into CSF,
	4th Vent
		Activity: "PEcK" and
		• *H. influenzae* }
		• *Enterobacter* } "HENPEcK"
		• *Neisseria* }
		
		NEVER use in CSF (IT)
		• except CEFUROXIME
		  against *H. influenzae*
		• others NOT effective
		
		CEFOXITIN – 1° against
		anaerobes (*Bacteroides*)
			Better against:
			1. *Enterobacter*
			  • Most stable to β-lactamase
			2. *Pseudomonas*
			  • CEFTAZIDIME
			  • CEFTRIAXONE
			3. Active: "HENPEcK" +
			  • *Pseudomonas* } "PHENPEcKS"
			  • *Serratia* }
			
			Adequate CSF Levels
			• Tx: meningitis
			• 1st and 2nd generation can NOT
			• 3rd Gen: *H. influenzae* meningitis
			  CEFOTAXIME, CEFTRIAXONE
			
			CEFTRIAXONE:
			1. D.O.C. – PENase producing
			  Neisseria
			2. *H. influenzae* meningitis – CSF
			3. Urinary tract infection
			4. Excreted in bile

Increased Activity to Gram (-), Decreased Activity to Gm(+), Increased Resistance to β-Lactamase →

GENERAL PROPERTIES OF CEPHALO-SPORINS

STRUCTURE
1. β-lactam ring and a 6 membered ring
2. Resistant to *Staph* PENase
3. Susceptible to • acid hydrolysis
   • β-lactamase
4. R_1 substitution: Δ bacterial spectrum
   • Δ β-lactamase susceptibility
   • Δ host toxicity
5. R_2 substitution – Δ kinetics

MECHANISM OF ACTION
Same as PENICILLIN
• β-lactam inhibits peptidoglycan
Resistance mechanism – same

DISTRIBUTION
$T_{1/2}$ = 30 min, all need multiple dosing
• Except: CEFTRIAXONE $\}$ $T_{1/2}$ = 6 hr
  CEFONICID
Bound to plasma proteins
Distributed well
Do NOT enter CNS unless INFLAMED
NEVER use 1st or 2nd generation
  CEPHS for meningitis
MENINGITIS Use 3rd generation drugs
CEFOTAXIME, CEFTRIAXONE,
(CEFUROXIME (2nd Gen) -*H. influenzae*)

BONE / OSTEOMYELITIS
CEFAZOLIN (1st Gen)
CEFTIZOXIME (3rd Gen)

BILIARY TRACT
CEFOPERAZONE (3rd Gen)
CEFTRIAXONE (3rd Gen)
CEFAMANDOLE (2nd Gen)

URINARY TRACT INFECTIONS (UTI)
CEFOPERAZONE (3rd)
CEFTRIAXONE (3rd)
ALL can cross the placenta

METABOLISM

$$R_1 - N \overset{S}{\underset{N}{\bigcirc}} O - R_2$$

Hydrolysis
• some metabolites have activity

EXCRETION
1. Kidney: glomerular filtration, secretion
   PROBENECID
   Does NOT Inc conc in some cases
2. Biliary: CEFAMANDOLE (2nd)
   CEFOPERAZONE (3rd)
   CEFTRIAXONE (3rd)
   High Conc in bile – use if renal impaired

SIDE EFFECTS
1. Allergy • Hypersensitivity
   • 15% cross react with PEN
2. More Nephrotoxic –
   CEPHALOTHIN + GENTAMICIN
3. Antibiotic-induced colitis
4. DISULFIRAM reaction: alcohol ingested
   Drug inhibits alcohol dehydrogenase
   • CEFAMANDOLE (2nd)
   • CEFOPERAZONE (3rd)
   • MOXALACTAM (3rd)
5. Bleeding – Vit K supplement needed
   • CEFAMANDOLE (2nd)
   • CEFOPERAZONE (3rd)
   • MOXALACTAM (3rd)
6. Thrombophlebitis – CEPHALOTHIN

CEFIXIME

• (3rd) (Oral)
• More like a 2nd Gen CEPH
  in spectrum
• Can NOT be used for
  Bacteremia or *Pseudomonas*

PENICILLIN SUBSTITUTES NON β-LACTAMS	ERYTHROMYCIN [237]
MODE OF ACTION	BACTERIOCIDAL or STATIC Depends on density, species of bacteria, & conc of antibiotic Macrolide – large lactone ring with 2 sugars • One of the safest drugs • Unstable in acid Inhibits protein synth by binding to 50 S ribosomal subunit • Binding site is close to that of: CHLORAMPHENICOL CLINDAMYCIN / LINCOMYCIN • Affects translocation • Interferes with peptidoglycan
RESISTANCE	Absence of receptors • NOT taken up Dec affinity for 50 S subunit • Δ in 23 S subunit – dimethylated Esterase – hydrolyzes antibiotic
SPECTRUM	(Like PEN G) • *Strep.* (NOT *viridans*) • *S. aureus* USES 1. D.O.C . – Mycoplasma Pneumonia 2. *Legionella* (IV) 3. *C. diphtheria* 4. UTI: *Chlamydia* and *Ureaplasma* 5. Gastroenteritis: *C. jejuni, Helicobacter, G. pneumocci* Use if allergic to PENICILLIN G
ADMINISTRATION	Oral • free base, stearate, estolate, ethyl succinate IV • lactobionate, gluceptate • thrombophlebitis IM • pain
DISTRIBUTION	Good penetration into body fluids Increases with inflammation • Except CNS – even with inflammation • All forms absorbed • Good level • Pulmonary fluids • Accumulate in MØ and PMN • Concentrate in liver • Cross placenta
EXCRETION	Conc and metab (P_{450}) in liver, excreted in bile, feces – enterohepatic recirculation. 10% into urine – enough to Tx: UTI
SIDE EFFECTS TOXICITY	DRUG INTERACTIONS Warfarin (Inc PT), Cyclosporine, Carbamazepine, Methylprednisolone, Theophylline, Digoxin; (Inc toxicity) 1. Epigastric distress – with ILOSONE® Cholestatic jaundice – Dec bile flow 2. Transient Deafness 3. Contraindicated w/ hepatic dysfunction 4. Superinfection – *Candida* GI, vagina 5. Inhibit metab: Theophylline, Digoxin, Cyclosporine, Carbamezepine, Methylprednisolone

VANCOMYCIN[238]	LINCOMYCIN[239] CLINDAMYCIN

BACTERIOCIDAL
  Complex, soluble, glycopeptide
 	
Inhibits cell wall synthesis at
  • phospholipids as well as peptidoglycan
  • NOT at transpeptidation step
Requires organism with PG cell wall
Most effective during growth phase
	BACTERIOSTATIC or CIDAL
	CLIND is the Cl analog of LINCOMYCIN
	
	Inhibits protein synthesis by binding to 50
	S ribosomal subunit
	  • Binding site is close to that of:
	  CHLORAMPHENICOL, ERYTHROMYCIN
	Inhibits peptidyl transferase

(Same as for PENICILLIN)
  • Absence of PG from cell wall
  • NOT degraded by enzymes
	Some cross resistance – ERYTHROMYCIN
	  • NO esterase cleavage
	  • Adenylation – dimethyl 23 S subunit

Very narrow spectrum (Like PEN G)
Staph. aureus (PEN Resistant),
Staph. epidermidis, Streptococcus,
Clostridium tetani and *C. diptheriae,*
N. gonorrhoeae, Enterococci
USES
1. D.O.C.: MRSA (If don't have, try
  CIPROFLOXACIN)
2. *Clostridium difficile* or *Staph. colitis*
3. *C. diphtheriae* endocarditis
  – use VANCO + AMINOGLYCOGEN
4. PEN allergic Pt – prophylaxis, dental
	Like PEN G – a substitute
	Also treat:
	  • Anaerobes (*Bacteroides fragilis*)
	  – CLINDAMYCIN
	  • *Staph* osteomyelitis – LINCOMYCIN
	  • *C. difficile* – Pseudomem colitis
	
	NOT effective against:
	  • Gm (-) aerobes – Enterobacteria
	  • Gm (+) anaerobes

NOT effective orally (unless *C. difficile*)
Oral → GI Tx   IV → systemic Tx
IV: Intermittent infusion 1 hr
  • Rapid histamine release – shock
  • Vasodilates, Red Man reaction
	CLINDAMYCIN:
	Oral: Well absorbed
	  IV: Improved absorption
	LINCOMYCIN: IV – thrombophlebitis

Good penetration into body fluids
  • Pericardial, pleural, synovial fluids
  • Penetrate CNS if inflamed but NOT
    adequate: give IT (intrathecal)
	Same as ERYTHROMYCIN
	  • Into fluids and bone, crosses placenta
	  • NOT CNS – even with inflammation
	    (CHLORAMPHENICOL – into CNS)
	  • Extensive metabolism (P_{450}) – dimethyl
	    potent antibacterial agent

Excreted unchanged by kidney – filtration
  • Normal $T_{1/2}$ = 6 – 8 hr
  • Anuric $T_{1/2}$ = 9 days (adjust dose)
	Activity seen in bile and urine
	  • Urine conc NOT high enough for Tx: UTI
	  • Glomerular filtration insignificant

1. Fast IV – Hypotension, shock – phlebitis
  at infusion site
2. Fever – chills
3. Allergies: rash with chronic use
4. Ototoxicity: CN VIII damage (irreversible)
5. Nephrotoxicity
	Renal failure: NO need to adjust dose
	Liver failure: Very Important to adjust
	    the dose

BACITRACIN[240]
  • Inhibits cell wall synthesis
  • Gram (-) organisms
  • Topical because nephrotoxic
	1. Nausea, vomiting, diarrhea
	  • persists in the GI tract – colitis
	2. Too rapidly • Hypotensive crisis
	            • Cardiovascular collapse
	3. Pseudo colitis • DON'T give antidiarrheal
	  • Give: VANCOMYCIN, BACITRACIN or
	    METRONIDAZOLE
	4. Potentiates neuromuscular blocking
	5. Very rare hepatotoxicity

BROAD-SPECTRUM ANTIBIOTICS	CHLORAMPHENICOL [241]
	Nitrobenzene derivative with 2 chlorines, 2 chiral centers, 4 Isomers, 1 active – Good, but very toxic
MECHANISM OF ACTION	Same as ERYTHROMYCIN and CLINDAMYCIN • Binds the 50 S subunit • Inhibits peptidyl transferase NOT effective against 80 S ribosomes (mammalian) • But mitochondrial 70 S ribosomes are suspect at high conc
RESISTANCE	R factor – acetylates drug in some organisms (AcCoA transferase) Inability to penetrate organism –Typhoid epidemic and *Shigella*
	BACTERIOCIDAL or STATIC – Depends upon the organism
SPECTRUM	*H. influenza* – meningitis, epiglottitis (Today use: CEFTRIAXONE or CEFOTAXIME) Anaerobic abscess in the brain Typhoid, *Rickettsia*, anaerobes (*B. fragilis*)
ABSORPTION	Oral: Absorbed very well – Very fat soluble IV: monosuccinate – ester
DISTRIBUTION	Excellent penetration everywhere • CNS without inflammation • Into abscesses
METABOLISM **EXCRETION**	Metab: Extensive – conjugation with glucuronic acid – inactive if hepatic failure: Problem with glucuronidation (low in neonates). Chloramphenicol oxamyl chloride – Inhibits P_{450} (interacts). Potentiates: Warfarin, Tolbutamide, Phenytoin, Coumadin 　[Any drug that Inc P_{450} activity (PHENOBARB, RIFAMPIN) will dec the $T_{1/2}$ of CHLORAMPHENICOL] Excretion depends on glucuronide formation (90%) Renal failure – glucuronide accumulates – NO need to Δ dose
SIDE EFFECTS **TOXICITY**	1. Hemolytic anemia • G-6-P DH deficiency (Mediterranean) 2. Reversible (toxic) anemia • dose related 3. Aplastic anemia • irreversible, NOT dose related, fatal

	TOXIC ANEMIA	ANAPLASTIC
a. Marrow	Normocellular	Hypo / Aplastic
b. Periph Blood	Anemia w/wo Leukopenia	Pancytopenia
c. Dose Related	Yes	No
d. Concomitant with Tx	Yes	No
e. Presenting	Anemia, Dec Hb Inc Serum Fe	Purpura Hemorrhage
f. Duration	Reversible	Irreversible

4. Gray Baby Syndrome – Neonate can't metabolize as well
　Dec feeding, vomiting, cyanosis, death
5. Children with early Tx: Inc incidence of ALL

TETRACYCLINE [242]	
CHLORTETRACYCLINE, DEMECLOCYCLINE, DOXYCYCLINE, MINOCYCLINE	
Must be taken up by energy-dependent transport system • NOT found in mammalian cells Acid stable • Binds 30 S subunit • Blocks access to amino acyl tRNA • Blocks protein synthesis	MECH OF ACTION
Common problem – Overused: Staph & some Strep resistant Change in uptake ability Accelerated efflux of drugs Cross resistance between all TETRACYCLINES	RESISTANCE
BACTERIOSTATIC	
Rickettsiae, Mycoplasma pneumonia, Lyme disease, *Chlamydia* – psittacosis, trachoma, lymphogranuloma venereum Acne vulgaris – Dec fatty acid synthesis in the skin Intestinal forms of amebiasis *Vibrio cholerae, Brucella* MINOCYCLINE – Tx: meningococcal carrier state	SPECTRUM
Oral: Absorbed well • Dec absorption with Ca^{++} and antacids (Mg^{++}) • Teeth and bone deposits – Temporary arrest of bone growth • Ca^{++} and Al^{+++} chelate TETRACYCLINES • Acid (Low pH) – Inc absorption • BICARB – Dec systemic amount, more stable	ABSORPTION
Does NOT get into CSF well – except MINOCYCLINE (Inflamed) All get into placenta → Inc in conc, fetal tissue • Conc in liver and kidney	DISTRIBUTION

1. DOXYCYCLINE → liver → glucuronidation → bile → feces
2. All others: glucuronide → reabsorbed, excreted in urine
  Kidney failure: – accumulate glucuronides
              – only use DOXYCYCLINE
	METABOLISM
	
	EXCRETION

1. GI Distress (Take with non-dairy foods to reduce) 2. Deposition in bone and 1° dentition (avoid in children < 8 yr) 3. Phototoxicity: DIMETHYCHLOR and DOXYCYCLINE a. sunburn b. onycholysis (nails come off nail beds) 4. Fatal hepatotoxicity: pregnant female with pyelonephritis 5. Vestibular problem: dizziness, endolymph (MINOCYCLINE) 6. Superinfection with yeast, *Candida* – vagina; Staph – GI 7. Oral contraceptives: Less effective • Inhibits bacteria which hydrolyze conjugated estrogen 8. Fanconi syndrome: TETRACYC + ASCORBIC ACID • Reacts on itself → nephrotoxic compound	SIDE EFFECTS TOXICITY

AMINOGLYCOSIDES [243]

STREPTOMYCIN ⎫
NEOMYCIN ⎪ _Streptomyces_
KANAMYCIN ⎬ species
TOBRAMYCIN ⎭

AMIKACIN – Acetylated KANAMYCIN

GENTAMICIN ⎫ gram-negative
NETILMICIN ⎭ species

BACTERIOCIDAL

Used to be D.O.C. for many organisms, but toxic

Important in treatment of biliary infections

- Very water soluble
- Stable over a wide pH
- Biologically stable
- NOT metabolized _in vivo_
- Coprecipitates with Heparin
- Given in adjunct with β-Lactams, NEVER in same solution
- Aminocyclitol ring with 3 different amino sugars

EXAMPLE: STREPTOMYCIN MODE OF ACTION

Binds irreversibly to 30 S subunit

- Misreads the code
- Depletes the 30 S subunit pool
- Blocks binding of the 30 S with mRNA or tRNA
- Bacteriostatic and bacteriocidal

Other aminoglycosides bind 30 S, some bind 50 S

SPECTRUM

- *Aerobes – O_2 and energy-dependent uptake system
- Does NOT affect anaerobes (or _Bacteroides fragilis_)

RESISTANCE

1. NO uptake system (anaerobes)
2. Δ binding sites on 30 S
3. Plasmid R factors – enzyme inactivation
   3 types with many different specificities
   - Acetyl transferase
   - Nucleotidyltransferase
   - Phosphotransferase
   NOT much cross reactivity – resistance

SPECTRUM

STREPTOMYCIN

1. _M. tuberculosis_
2. Endocarditis – _S. viridans_ or enterococci
3. _Yersinia pestis_
4. _Vibrio cholerae_

GENTAMICIN and TOBRAMYCIN

1. Aerobic Gm (-) (_Enterobacter, E. coli_)
2. _Pseudomonas_

AMIKACIN (Only if resistant to GENTAMICIN / TOBRAMYCIN)

1. Aerobic Gm (-) (_Enterobacter, E. coli_)
2. _Pseudomonas_

SYNERGISTIC with β-Lactams (PENs and CEPHs)

- Interact with each other
- Inactivate – toxic if in same solution

CLINICAL INDICATIONS
EMPIRIC

Neonatal sepsis
Nosocomial pneumonia
Febrile episode in granulopenic host
Biliary tract sepsis
Intraabdominal

DEFINITIVE

Pseudomonal infection
Enterococci infection
S. aureus
P. aeruginosa
Transurethral resection of prostate

AMINOGLYCOSIDES [243]

PHARMACOLOGY
NOT Oral – Not absorbed well
  (except NEOMYCIN)
IV or IM only
Loading dose to start – IV slowly

NEOMYCIN – oral (exception)
• Topical or oral (NOT IV, IM, IT)
• Sterilize the gut for bowel surgery
• Hepatic coma – Dec NH_4
• Does NOT bind protein – negligible

DISTRIBUTION
Extracellular fluid volume
• Distrib is NOT good, poorly distrib
• Low binding, Dec Vol Distrib
• Except ear and kidney – high conc

GENTAMICIN, TOBRAMYCIN and
  AMIKACIN
• Obese – Dec ECF → Inc serum [ ]
• Fever – Dec ECF → Inc serum [ ]
• Edema – Inc ECF → Dec serum [ ]

Does NOT get into the CNS
• IT (Intrathecal)
• Intraventricularly
  (Except NEOMYCIN – Do NOT use it)

Bronchial fluid – 20% serum value
• Does NOT get into Pulm system well

EAR and KIDNEY – high levels

All cross the placenta

GENTAMICIN, TOBRAMYCIN, and
  NETILMICIN
4 – 10 µg/ml – therapeutic dose
> Conc is nephrotoxic

AMIKACIN – Better therapeutic range
4 – 35 µg/ml dose

NO metabolic inactivation
Humans can't metabolize AmGly
Only bacteria can

EXCRETION
Kidney – rapidly into urine

Azotemia – Dec creatinine clearance
Inc the $T_{1/2}$ (Dec dose)
Always check the blood
$T_{1/2}$ = 2 hrs (quick)
Anuric = 50 – 100 hrs
Neonate = 5 – 6 hrs

ACCUMULATES IN
1. Renal cortex – nephrotoxic
2. Endolymph – ototoxic
3. Perilymph – ototoxic

SIDE EFFECTS
1. Renal disease
2. Ototoxicity – Reacts with hair cell organ
   of Corti, lose high tones first
   a. Cochlea – KANAMYCIN
                AMIKACIN
                NEOMYCIN
                – Deafness, tinnitus, dizziness
   b. Vestibule – STREPTOMYCIN
                  GENTAMICIN
                  TOBRAMYCIN
                  NETILMICIN

TOXICITY
Binds to phosphatidyl inositol in ear and
kidney – PCT necrosis
3. Neuromuscular paralysis
   – Do NOT give as bolus injection
4. Allergic skin reaction – NEOMYCIN

INTERACTIONS / CONTRAINDICATIONS
1. GENTAMICIN + CEPHALOTHIN
   TOBRAMYCIN + CEPHALOTHIN
   – Inc nephrotoxicity
2. FUROSEMIDE + AMINOGLYCOSIDE
   ETHACRYNIC ACID + AMINOGLYCOSIDE
   • Inc ototoxicity
3. AMINOGLYCOSIDE + HEPARIN
   • coprecipitates

NEPHROTOXICITY
NEO > GENTA > TOBRA > AMIKACIN

DO NOT UNDERDOSE
• Delays recovery
• Can worsen
• Inc risk of complication

TUBERCULOSIS CHEMOTx	1° TREATMENT	
	ISONIAZID [244]	RIFAMPIN [245]
MODE OF ACTION	BACTERIOCIDAL • Dec DNA synthesis • Dec mycolic acid synthesis • Minor MAO inhibitor • Enhances permeability of other drugs against TB	BACTERIOCIDAL • BROAD SPECTRUM Inhibits DNA dependent RNA synthesis • Suppresses chain initiation and transcription Higher affinity for bacterial enzymes Oral – well absorbed
RESISTANCE	Inability to uptake and concentrate	Binds Subunit β' $\Delta \beta'$ • Dec affinity
TB SPECTRUM	Very narrow spectrum *M. tuberculosis* Only (NOT atypicals) – Prophylaxis & Tx	*M. tuberculosis* Atypical mycobacteria Staph – Can become resistant *Legionella* – resistant ERYTHROMYCIN Meningococcal meningitis MRSA Gm (-): *Klebsiella, E. coli, Shigella*
ADMINISTRATION ABSORPTION	Orally effective INH + RIF + PYRA, first 2 months INH + RIF , 4 months	Oral: lipid soluble
DISTRIBUTION	Total body water Penetrates caseous material • CNS (without inflammation) • Crosses placenta Tx: fetal bone, tooth, CNS defects	All Fluids • Urine, sweat, tears • Red/Orange color • CNS (without inflammation)
EXCRETION	Genetic – bimodal NAc transferase Rapid $T_{1/2}$ = 1.5 hr, Slow $T_{1/2}$ = 3 hr Acetylates INH • Hepatic disease • Dec dose • Age dependent	Liver – Enterohepatic circulation Deacetylated form • Still active • NOT recirculated $T_{1/2}$ = 1.5 - 5 hr Bile-dependent excretion
SIDE EFFECTS	Slow acetylators • Clear up faster • More drug interactions • Dec metabolism of: PHENYTOIN and oral anticoagulants 1. Periph neuropathy: Mito swell, retrograde, paresthesia (tingle), sensory loss, Inc Vit B_6 loss 2. CNS: dizzy, ataxia, Δ mood, psychosis, memory loss, disulfiram reaction 3. Convulsions 4. Hepatic failure 5. Hemolytic anemia G-6-P DH deficit 6. Hypersensitivity – rash	1. GI upset (eat) 2. Asymptomatic Inc liver enzyme 3. Hepatotoxic 4. Allergies – Ab – fever, chills – myalgia 5. Eosinophilia 6. Interstitial nephritis Induces P_{450} Inc metab of other drugs → Dec: • CONTRACEPTIVES • ANTICOAGULANTS • KETOCONAZOLE • DIGITOXIN • METHADONE IV Drug Users • CHLORAMPHENICOL

1° TREATMENT		2° TREATMENT	
PYRAZINAMIDE [246]	**ETHAMBUTOL** [247]	**STREPTOMYCIN** [248]	**OTHER 2°** [249]
BACTERIOCIDAL Hepatotoxic Unknown mechanism	BACTERIOSTATIC Requires growing organism Interferes with DNA and protein synthesis Use INH, RIF, and ETHAM in patients with HIV and TB	Binds irreversibly to 30 S subunit • Inhibits protein synthesis IV, NOT active orally Aminoglycoside	Para- AMINO SALICYLATE (PAS) ETHIONAMIDE CYCLOSERINE AMIKACIN KANAMYCIN Poorly STATIC Need high quantities
	Resistance develops slowly compared to RIFAMPIN		Inhibit incorporation of PABA into folate
M. tuberculosis Requires acidic environment (in MØ)	*M. tuberculosis* • For INH + RIF resistant organisms • Atypicals • Resistant strains	If resistant to other drugs	Only *Mycobacterium*
Orally active	Oral	Parenterally, IM	CYCLOSERINE • Liver damage • Peripheral neuropathy
Penetrates cells well	In CNS when inflamed Conc in RBCs	Polar Does NOT penetrate cells or caseous material	PAS: • Granulocytopenia • Interfere with RIFAMPIN • Bacteriostatic • GI disturbance • Allergic rash • Similar PABA • Inhibits folate synthesis • Fever • Joint pain
	Renal excretion		
One metabolite • Prevents uric acid secretion • Precipitates gout arthritis Nausea, vomiting, arthralgia, fever Exacerbates diabetes Hepatotoxic	Retrobulbar neuritis • Dec visual acuity • CANNOT distinguish red / green Generally safe •Inc plasma urate → Gout	Ototoxic – vestibule Nephrotoxic (like all aminoglycosides)	ETHIONAMIDE • Very toxic • GI disturbance • Liver damage • Periph neuropathy • Optic neuritis KANAMYCIN AMIKACIN • Aminoglycoside • Must give IV • Ototoxic (VIII) • Nephrotoxic • GI disturbances

TUBERCULOSIS

Natural Resistance
1. Mycolic acid
2. Slow growth rate

ANTIFUNGAL	AMPHOTERICIN B [250]	FLUCYTOSINE [251]
MODE OF ACTION	Polyene antibiotic Lipophilic and polar groups Forms pores in fungi • 8 molecules – pore • Most toxic • Inc permeability – lose contents • Selectively bind ergosterols • AMP B + FLU – synergistic Systemic infection	5 fluorouracil • 5 Fl UMP – active • Inhibits DNA synthesis dUMP → dTMP Inhibits NA formation • Pyrimidine analog Systemic infections • Amp B + FLU
RESISTANCE	Dec ergosterol concentration of fungal membrane	NOT given alone Resistance develops Δ PERMEASE Δ DEAMINASE AMP B adjunct • together Dec dose → Dec toxicity
SPECTRUM	FUNGICIDAL, some amoebae, NOT for *E.histolytica* • Disseminated or miliary disease • D.O.C.: Pulm infection (except blastomycosis – KETOKONAZOLE)	Cryptococcal meningitis *Candida albicans*
ADMINISTRATION	Not oral – IV, slowly • Binds to lipoprotein • Does NOT penetrate CNS • IT – Cryptococcal meningitis • NOT stable in solution 5% dextrose only Tx: 4 – 6 months	Oral • Penetrates CNS • Cryptococcal meningitis
DISTRIBUTION	LIPO and HYDROPHILIC Polar cap – acidic	Penetrates CNS
EXCRETION	Urine Monitor creatinine for toxicity To avoid problems, hydrate well	Depends on renal function
SIDE EFFECTS	50%: Chills, fever, vomiting (prevent with steroids) 80%: Some renal damage, mild tubular acidosis, reversible nephrotoxicity (If > 4g – permanent toxicity) Hypokalemia – weakness Cardiac arrest Hypocellular glomerulus tubule degeneration, fibrosis Normochromic anemia Pain Chemical meningitis IT: pain, headache, painful micturition	Bone marrow depression • Anemia • Leukopenia • Thrombocytopenia GI Upset • Enterocolitis Elevated Hepatic Enzyme

KETOCONAZOLE [252]	GRISEOFULVIN [253]	NYSTATIN [254]
Imidazole BACTERIOSTATIC • Dec ergosterol synthesis • Interferes with P_{450} yeast • Leaky cell → dies Similar to sterols Systemic and dermal	Binds tubulin of mitotic spindle • Interferes with cell division • Metaphase arrest Clears infection from inside out Dermatophyte infections	Polyene antibiotic Oral, vaginal, GI candidiasis Topical Oral lozenge NOT absorbed
Limited use with immuno- compromised patients AMP B + KETO – Bad Effect Inhibit Each Other		CANDICIDIN (polyenes) Binds sterols and forms pores like AMP B
• D.O.C. *Paracoccidioides* • Simple Pulm blastomycosis • Chronic mucocutaneous vaginitis • Prophylaxis and treatment	Dermatophylic infections • Superficial lesions • Given systemically • Energy-dependent absorption	Oral – GI candidiasis Too toxic parenteral
Oral: adequate acid solution • Systemic infection • Solution – highly acidic NOT IV or IM: acid necrosis • NOT buffered • H_2 blocker – inactivates Dec HCl secretion	Binds keratin, as new layer moves out, infection clears Duration Tx – long Parenterally Lipid soluble Inc absorption with a fatty meal	OTHERS: TOLNAFTATE – O.T.C. Topical, dermatophytes UNDECYLENIC ACID • Cruex® • Unsaturated fatty acid CANDICIDIN
Does NOT go into CNS Mostly bound to plasma proteins Distributes in: synovial, saliva, milk, vaginal secretions	Oral: Inhibits (non topical) derm fungi NOT destroyed by topical agents Water insoluble NOT absorbed well Micronized powder	
Extensive metabolism Excreted by kidney as inactive form ∴ NOT useful for UTI Elimination: dose-dependent $200 mg T_{1/2} = 1.5 hr$ $800 mg T_{1/2} = 4 hr$		FLUCONAZOLE (DIFLUCAN®) • New – less sterol SE's • NO gynecomastia • NO loss of libido • NO menstrual Δ
Well tolerated Epigastric pain Nausea, vomiting – dose depend, Anorexia, headache Photophobia Peripheral neuritis Gynecomastia – steroid effect Menstrual irregularity Loss of libido Inc liver enzymes Blunt adrenal response to ACTH Dec metabolism CYCLOSPORINE A Inc immunosuppression Fungal infection worsens	Headache, confusion, fatigue, ataxia, Potentiated by alcohol GI: nausea, pain Rare Allergies: • angioedema • serum sickness Induces mixed function Ox oral anticoagulant Precipitates acute porphyria Contraindicated: • Pregnancy (fetal toxic) • Porphyria Cross sensitive with Penicillin allergies	TYPES OF FUNGI 1. SYSTEMIC • *Blastomyces* • *Histoplasma* • *Sporotrichosis* • *Coccidioides* • *Paracoccidioides* • *Cryptococcus* 2. CANDIDIASIS 3. DERMATOPHYTE • *Microsporum* • *Trichophyton* • *Epidermophyton*

ANTIVIRAL AGENTS	ACYCLOVIR [255]	GANCICLOVIR [256]
MODE OF ACTION	Against DNA viruses Acyclo-GTP (active) 1. Inhibits DNA polymerase 2. Incorporates into viral DNA terminates DNA synthesis Specific for herpes virus thymidine kinase	Like ACYCLOVIR
RESISTANCE	Dec viral coded thymidine kinase	
VIRAL SPECTRUM	HSV 1 and 2 – genitals – keratitis Varicella–zoster virus D.O.C.: Herpes encephalitis – cure NOT effective against cytomegalovirus *Herpes genitalis* – NO cure, relieve symptoms	Active against herpes including cyto-megalovirus (CMV) • Use with liver & kidney transplant No effect on HIV
ADMINISTRATION ABSORPTION	Topical: keratitis – NO cure Oral: genitals – NO cure IV: encephalitis – cure	
DISTRIBUTION	Penetrates well Penetrates CNS D.O.C.: herpetic encephalitis $T_{1/2}$ = 2.5 hr	
EXCRETION	Kidney Monitor renal function disease $T_{1/2}$ = 20 hr	

SIDE EFFECTS	Topical: burning, irritation
	IV: Slowly – hypotensive shock
	
	Nausea, vomiting – centrally
	Bone marrow suppression
	  Leukopenia
	  Thrombocytopenia
	
	CNS depression
	  Lethargy, vertigo, sedation, coma
	
	CNS stimulation
	  Seizure, tremors
	
	Transient renal dysfunction
	  If hydrate – OK	

VIDARABINE [257]	AMANTADINE [258]	[259] AZIDOTHYMIDINE ZIDOVUDINE (AZT)	[260] IDOXURIDINE
Inhibits viral DNA polymerase Purine analog	Interferes with viral uncoating Can NOT penetrate cells	Inhibits retroviruses' reverse transcriptase Inhibits viral replication NOT a cure for AIDS	
D.O.C.: Herpes keratitis and conjunctivitis	1. Prophylaxis of Asian A$_2$ virus – All strains At risk: • Elderly epidemics • Very young with pulmonary problems 2. Parkinsonism	HIV: Dec morbidity & mortality Inc survival time Dec 2° infections (*P. carinii*) NOT a cure	Topical Tx of herpetic keratitis and conjunctiva
Topical Systemic	Oral		
		Crosses blood brain barrier into CNS Tx: encephalitis	
CNS effects • Hallucinations Systemic side effects • Mutagenic • Carcinogenic Topically • NO side effects	Interferes with drug metabolism • Anticoagulants High dose: CNS Effects 1. Ataxia 2. Confusion 3. Lethargy 4. Depression 5. Seizures	Bone marrow suppression (myelo-suppression)	VERY TOXIC NOT used now Use VIDARABINE

ANTIMALARIAL DRUGS	PRIMAQUINE[261]	QUININE[262]
MODE OF ACTION	Dec energy production in sensitive organisms Mitochondria swell NO correlation between plasma level and effect Metabolites probably active Casual prophylaxis Exoerythrocytic form only Opposite of CHLOROQUINE	
RESISTANCE	Develops slowly – rare Tx: *P. vivax, P. malariae* Prophylaxis of *P. falciparum* NOT effective Tx: *P. falciparum*	

ANTIMALARIAL SPECTRUM	Only EXOERYTHROCYTIC
	– tissue (liver) schizonticide
	GAMETOCYTOCIDAL, too
	2° Exoerythrocytic
	   P. vivax
	   P. ovale
		CHLOROQ resistant strains
		EXOERYTHROCYTIC stage only
		Curare-like effect
		Tx: Nocturnal leg cramps

ADMINISTRATION	Oral: well absorbed Not concentrated (like CHLOROQ) 2 doses / day Therapeutic Index: 10 Safe	Oral IV
DISTRIBUTION		
EXCRETION	Extensively metabolized – Liver Rapid metabolism $T_{1/2}$ is short	Urine
SIDE EFFECTS	IV: Dec BP°, Δ ECG, Heart Effects Oral: 1. Hemolytic anemia • G-6-P DH 2. Aggravates Systemic Lupus Erythematosus 3. Abdominal cramps 4. Epigastric distress 5. Methemoglobinemia CONTRAINDICATED • Granulocytosis • Lupus (SLE) • Rheumatoid arthritis (Note – Opposite of CHLOROQ)	More toxic than PRIMAQUINE CARDIOTOXIC • Cardiac depression • Ventricular fibrillation • Δ ECG • Hypotensive shock – vasodilation CHINCONISM • Tinnitus • Deafness • Headaches • Visual disturbances Curare-like effect Potentiates myasthenia gravis

SULFADOXINE PYRIMETHAMINE (Fansidar®) [263]	CHLOROQUINE [264]	MEFLOQUINE [265]

Inhibits dihydrofolate reductase
• Dec dihydrofolate
	Intercalates with DNA
	Dec synthesis of DNA & RNA
	Δ DNA melting point
	SELECTIVE TOXICITY
	  1. CHLOROQ is a base – acid
	    environment of infected RBC
	  2. Uptake active transport
	  Schizonticidal
	  Opposite of PRIMAQUINE
		Unknown

Develops rapidly (during therapy) and passes resistance onto the next generation	Inc efflux of the drug (some cancers, too) Dec $T_{1/2}$ (2 min)	

ERYTHROCYTIC GAMETOCIDAL
 	
Also, Tx: TOXOPLASMOSIS
	D.O.C.: acute malaria
	  ERYTHROCYTIC only
	
	Other uses:
	  1. Extraintestinal amoeba
	  2. Antiinflammatory prophylaxis
	    and Tx: a. Rheumatoid arthritis
	          b. SLE
		Reserved for multiresistant organisms
		
		ERYTHROCYTIC Only

	Orally active Once a week Completely absorbed Concentrated in RBC	Oral
	Penetrates cells well Spleen, liver, kidney $T_{1/2}$ = 7 days	
Rapidly eliminated		$T_{1/2}$ = 14 days Single dose Long duration

Megaloblastic anemia (Give folic acid) Folate deficiency	Usually safe
	Problems with high doses
	  1. GI: nausea, vomiting
	  2. Cardiac arrest
	    Δ ECG – Dec T-wave
	  3. Eye – accumulates
	    • Corneal clouding
	    • Dec visual acuity
	    • Diplopia
	CONTRAINDICATED:
	  1. Pregnancy – fetal Δ
	  2. Psoriasis
	  3. Porphyria
		Mild GI upset

ANTIPROTOZOAL DRUGS	(LUMINAL) DILOXANIDE FUROATE [266]	DIIODOHYDROXYQUIN [267]
MODE OF ACTION	Unknown	
RESISTANCE		
USES	D.O.C.: Luminal amebiasis	Luminal amebiasis only
ADMINISTRATION **ABSORPTION**	Oral: • Split into DILOXANIDE and DILOXANIDE FUROATE • 90% absorbed – inactive • Glucuronide conjugated • 10% unabsorbed, active form	Oral: NOT absorbed
EXCRETION		
SIDE EFFECTS	Nausea, cramps, flatulence	

	TETRACYCLINE [268] PAROMOMYCIN	HALOGENATED [269] HYDROXYQUINOLINE IODOQUINOL, CLIOQUINOL
LEISHMANIASIS [270] • Na STIBOGLUCONATE • AMPHOTERICIN B • METRONIDAZOLE • ALLOPURINOL • NIFURTIMOX	• Aminoglycoside antibiotics • Amebicidal, also • NOT absorbed in GI • NOT toxic • Tx: Mild intestinal amebiasis	• Antiluminal • Serious side effects NOT used • GI disturbances • Interferes with thyroid CLIOQUINOL • Subacute neuropathy • Weak eye muscles • Visual Δ

| TRYPANOSOMIASIS
 1. African (*T. brucei*)
 • PENTAMIDINE
 • STILBAMIDINE
 • PROPAMIDINE
 Interferes with glucose utilization & binding of DNA | SIDE EFFECTS
 1. Hypotension
 2. Resp depression
 3. Nephro & neurotoxicity | 2. *T. cruzi*
 • NIFURTIMOX
 • Oxygen radicals
 SIDE EFFECTS
 • GI disturbances
 • Peripheral neuropathy |

(SYSTEMIC)	
METRONIDAZOLE (Flagyl®) [271]	**EMETINE** [272]
Anaerobic or microaerobic 1. Electron sink – interferes with energy production 2. Metabolite interferes w/ DNA synthesis – nick/break strand Nitrogen group reduced – amine Interferes with DNA replication	Interferes with protein synthesis Irreversible inhibition – translocation step Inhibits protein synthesis – elongation
NOT effective against carrier state	
D.O.C.: *T. vaginalis, E. histolytic,* Systemic ameba, *G. lamblia* Anaerobic bacteria Gram (+,-) • *C. perfringes* and *difficile* • *Bacteroides fragilis* • *Fusobacterium* Especially CNS without inflammation • Broad spectrum anaerobic infections of the CNS	Extraintestinal amebiasis • Liver and brain abscesses • Directly lethal to amebae *E. histolytica,* only Tissue amebiasis
Oral: well absorbed One metabolite is active • Hydroxy Metab (65% active) • Glucuronide metabolites	NOT Oral or IV IM only – Accumulates in the liver
Urine - Red/Brown	Cleared slowly

Nausea, vomiting, anorexia
Cramps
Metallic taste
Epigastric distress
GI: overgrowth of *Candida*
Neurotoxic: dizziness, ataxia
Peripheral neuropathy – sensory
Disulfiram reaction – alcohol
– Inc acetaldehyde – toxic
Hemolytic anemia – G-6-P DH deficiency
Neutropenia – dyscrasias
 	
EXPERIMENTALLY (long use)
• Mutagenic / carcinogenic
• NOT seen in humans
 	
CONTRAINDICATED
1. 1st Trimester pregnancy
2. History of blood dyscrasias
3. Neurologic problems
	Oral: GI disturbances
	  Nausea, vomiting, diarrhea
	
	IV: Cardiotoxicity
	  Hypotension
	  Tachycardia
	  Δ ECG
	  Dyspnea
	  Pain
	  Cardiac dilation – failure, death
	
	NEUROMUSCULAR EFFECTS
	Weakness, tender, flu-like, stiff neck
	Patients must be sitting
	
	CONTRAINDICATED
	1. Pregnancy
	2. Renal disease
	3. Neuromuscular problems
	4. Exercise – Inc EMETINE toxicity

7 OTHER TOPICS

PERINATAL PHARMACOLOGY

PHARMACODYNAMICS
Direct: Drug interacts directly with cells or tissue of fetus
Indirect: • Δ fetal environment
           • Δ blood delivery rate
           • Δ pH of blood

DIFFERENTIAL SUSCEPTIBILITY
By fetal developmental stage
1. Critical • during formation of organ systems
           • neural tube formation
           • palate fusion
2. Embryo may lack appropriate receptors until it develops them

DRUG EQUILIBRATION
1. Rapid between maternal blood and fetal blood
2. Slow between maternal blood and fetal tissues
        Example: THIOPENTAL • Mother quickly becomes unconscious
                                • Delay to fetus, spares baby – alert when born

PHARMACOKINETICS
1. Mother pH = 7.4, Fetal pH = 7.2
           • Ion trapping of weak basic drugs in fetal circulation
2. Umbilical vein → fetal circulation (like IV)
3. Fetus:
   a. Low albumin levels
           • Dec plasma protein binding
   b. Fetal liver – enzymes NOT as active
           • low metabolic capability
           • Dec first pass effect
   c. Blood shunted to upper body
   d. Water: fat ratio is greater in fetus
4. Excretion • umbilical artery
               • amniotic fluid is ingested
               • chronic exposure

> **FETAL ALCOHOL SYNDROME**
>
> 1. Small face
> 2. Small head
> 3. NO philtrum
> 4. Retarded behavior

FETAL ALCOHOL SYNDROME
• Mother drinks – fetus *in utero* experiences withdrawal
• Street drugs – CNS defects
• Fetal addiction

Breast feeding – source of exposure
Birthing drugs – controversial if prolonged birth
   e.g. Demerol® – fetal respiratory depression if birth takes 2 – 3 hrs

TOXICOLOGY [367] AIR POLLUTANTS	NITROGEN DIOXIDE (NO_2)	OZONE (O_3)	SULFUR DIOXIDE (SO_2)	CARBON MONOXIDE (CO)
	<u>SYMPTOMS</u> Local irritant of: • Eye • Upper respiratory tract • Stains skin and teeth <u>SYSTEMIC</u> • Pulmonary edema • Bronchiolar damage, life threatening obstruction • Methemoglobinemia 　MeHb REDase + NADPH 　Reduce $Fe^{+++} \rightarrow Fe^{++}$ • Choking • Lacrimation	$NO_2 - (UV) \rightarrow NO + O$ $O + O_2 \rightarrow O_3$ $NO + O_3 \rightarrow O_2 + NO_2$ 　in a clean environment $NO + HC \rightarrow NO_2 + Red HC$ 　in a polluted environment • Leaving O_3 (ozone) <u>SYMPTOMS</u> • Pulmonary edema • Δ Respiratory morphology • Inc lipid peroxidation • Histamine potentiates effect 　(anything that Inc ACh)	<u>SYMPTOMS</u> • Irritates nose, throat, and eyes • Lacrimation • Inc mucus, nose • Coughing, choking • Bronchoconstriction • Inc bronchial secretions • Inc pulmonary resistance • Rales • Bronchial asthma <u>SEVERE</u> • Chemical – bronchopneumonia	• Headache, dizziness • Nausea, vomiting, diarrhea • Loss of consciousness <u>CHRONIC POISONING</u> • Loss of muscle strength • Dec alertness • Persistent headaches • Light-headedness, dizziness • Auditory nerve damage

Poison – Any agent that can produce harm to living tissue
Pesticides – 3 Classes
  1. Chlorinated hydrocarbons
  2. Organic phosphates
  3. Dioxins
Dose dependent
LD_{50} by itself is NOT an accurate predictor of toxicity
Use other LDs also

GLUTATHIONE

• Protects body from free radicals
• If Glutathione is depleted METHIONINE is used

FOOD POLLUTANTS	SAXITOXIN [368]	FAVA BEAN	NITRATES [369]	ETHIONE AMIDE	GALACTOSAMINE	CARBON TETRACHLORIDE (CCl_4) [370]
	• Shellfish contaminant • Na^+ channel blocker	• Favism • 3,4 Di(OH)PHE • G-6-P DH deficiency → hemolytic anemia	Preservatives • Baby food Tx: Methylene blue • Oxidized form • IV	Liver metabolism Substitute into methionine Metab • Leads to cancer • Depletes ATP → fatty Δ liver	UTP for metabolism • Depletes uridine	Metab to CCl_3 • Cyto P 450 CCl_3 • Toxic • Tissue damage

WATER POLLUTANTS	CHLORINE			CHLORINE DIOXIDE		

	Past: Used to prevent cholera and typhoid
	Today: Reacts with industrial waste and insecticides to form carcinogens
	TRIHALOMETHANES
	CHLOROFORM $CH(Cl)_3$
	BROMODICHLOROMETHANE $CHBr(Cl)_2$
	DIBROMOCHLOROMETHANE $CH(Br)_2Cl$
	BROMOFORM $CH(Br)_3$
	IODOFORM
	Dose related: Inc liver, kidney, colon cancer
	U.S. limit of < 100 ppb in water
	  55 ppb Coca Cola (coloring)
	  7 ppb 7-Up, Sprite
	Hot shower – volatilize → inhale trihalomethanes
	Swimmers in chlorinated pools
	Seasonal – Inc during summer
				Alternative to chlorine
				• 5 x more potent
				• > 10 mg/L – crenated RBCs and dacryocysts
				• Powerful oxidizing agents
				• Stress the glutathione reductase system
				  G-6-P DH deficiency → hemolytic anemia		

TOXICOLOGY	TCDD [372]	MALATHION [373]	HEXANE [374]
	AGENT ORANGE contaminant	Organophosphate insecticide	• Neurotoxic
	• Defoliant	Pure: safe for human, toxic to insect	• Neuro atrophy
	50% 2,4 - dichlorophenoxyacetic acid	Cholinesterase	• Weakness, numbness
	50% 2,4,5 - trichlorophenoxyacetic acid	Metabolized in human:	peripheral → proximal
	1.9 ppm tetrachlorodibenzodioxin	• To harmless products by 2 enzymes:	• Pulmonary Δ
	• Dioxin contaminant	Carboxyesterase	• Death possible
		Glutathione alkyl transferase	
	__MECHANISM__	• Insects lack these enzymes	Mechanism:
	1. Penetrates liver cell membrane	Use Cyto P_{450}:	Metabolized by Cyto P_{450}
	2. Binds cytosolic receptors	MALATHION → MALAXON	hexane → 2-hexanone
	3. Enters nucleus → Δ mRNA	• MALAXON – ACh inhibitor	→ 2,5-hexadione
			• Inc toxicity as metabolized
	__EFFECTS__	Stored in heat → Isomalathion	
	1. Induces Cyto P_{450} in the liver:	• Isomal inhibits carboxyesterase	Methyl butyl ketone (MBK)
	(Reduces Cyto P_{450} in the adrenal gland)	• Uses Cyto P_{450} instead	= 2 hexanone
	Inc AHH (aryl hydrocarbon hydroxylase)	(as in the insect)	Methyl ethyl ketone (MEK)
	• AHH: benzoapyrine → carcinogen		• Induces Cyto P_{450}
	Inc ALA (alanine amino transferase)		• Potentiates MBK toxicity
	Inc GT (glutathione transferase)		
	Inc ornithine decarboxylase		
	2. Inhibits LDL metabolism		
	• Inc cholesterol synthesis		
	3. Inhibits 21 OHase (Progest → 11 DeOCort)		
	• Impairs spermatogenesis (Dec testosterone)		
	4. Dec corticosterone		
	Symptoms:		
	1. Rash 4. Weight loss		
	2. Neurologic Δ 5. Hydronephrosis		
	3. Teratogenic		

VOLATILE SOLVENTS 375	TOLUENE	XYLENE	ACETONE	BENZENE	GASOLINE	NAPHTHA	CCl₄	TRICHLOROETHYLENE
ACUTE TOXIC	Resp arrest Arrhythmias	Resp arrest Arrhythmias	Resp arrest Arrhythmias	Resp arrest Arrhythmias	Resp arrest Arrhythmias	Resp arrest Arrhythmias	Resp arrest Arrhythmias	
CHRONIC	Anemia Liver damage Kidney damage Brain damage Chromosomal damage			Leukemia Aplastic anemia Liver damage Kidney damage	Lead poisoning Liver damage		Liver damage	Neuropathy Liver damage Kidney damage

AEROSOLS	DEODORANTS	ASBESTOS	VINYL CHLORIDE	CHLORDECONE (KEPONE®) DIBROMOCHLOROPROPANE
Laryngospasms Airway freezing Suffocation Arrhythmia	Sarcoidosis	Lung cancer Mesothelioma	Liver cancer Latent 10 yrs	Insecticides • Sterility (males)

HEAVY METAL	LEAD (Pb) [376]	MERCURY (Hg) [377]
	Paint, putty, dirt, newsprint, industrial, plumbing, gasoline (organic)	Industrial, dental amalgams, fungicides, bacterial products

Lead Poisoning

EFFECTS
1. Hematopoietic System
   - Hypochromic, microcytic anemia
   - Inhibits heme synthesis / enzymes
   a. Aminolevulinic dehydratase
   b. Coproporphyrinogen oxidase
   c. Ferrochelatase
   - Inc Conc in urine of
   a. Amino levulinic acid
   b. Coproporphyrinogen
2. CNS: lead encephalopathy
   - Clumsy, irritable, Dec intelligence Dec consciousness, seizures, coma, death
   - If survive – retardation
3. Peripheral Nervous System
   - Weakness, paralysis, lead palsy, wrist drop, motor dysfunction, atrophy
4. Reproductive
   - Stillbirth, sterility, spontaneous abortion, neonatal death
5. GI Tract Δ – oral
   - GI spasm, abdominal pain

INORGANIC LEAD
Children: absorb 50%
Adults: absorb 10%
- 1° affects: blood system

ORGANIC LEAD
100% absorbed
- 1° affects: CNS system

LEAD ACCUMULATES
Soft Tissues: $T_{1/2}$ = 30 days
- liver, kidney, spleen
- Brain (organic)
Hard Tissues: $T_{1/2}$ = 20 – 30 years
- bone, teeth

Tx: Chelators
- DIMERCAPROL
- Ca EDTA
- PENICILLAMINE

INORGANIC EFFECTS
Acute: (GI)
- Nausea, vomiting, diarrhea, colitis, intestinal necrosis
- Renal shutdown

CHRONIC
CNS
- Tremor, ataxia, slurring, insomnia, mental deterioration
- Loose teeth
- Renal failure

ORGANIC
- Ataxia, tunnel vision, hearing loss, mental Δ, incoordination, paralysis, coma
- Renal failure

VAPOR
- Interstitial pneumonitis
- Pulmonary edema

PATHOLOGY
- Inhibits pyridine metabolism
- Blocks glucose transport
- Renal excretion

"Minimata" poisoning

Tx: PENICILLAMINE
DIMERCAPROL

CYANIDE (CN) [378]	CADMIUM (Cd) [379]	
Rapidly Fatal 1 - 2 min Binds Fe in ferric position (Fe^{+++}) Binds mitochondrial cytochrome oxidase → Histotoxic hypoxia Tx: 1. First give nitrite AMYL NITRITE (inhale) Na NITRITE (IV) • Δ Hb → MeHb • MeHb has Fe^{+++} • Competes for CN 2. Na THIOSULFATE • CN → Na ThioCN • Excreted in Urine 3. METHYLENE BLUE • MethHb → Hb	Plastics, paints, batteries, cigarettes, coal Acute: • Local irritation Chronic: • Renal injury • Pulmonary injury • Carcinogenic • Proteinuria • Inc aminolevulinic DH Tx: EDTA Dialysis • NOT effective	

> **ORGANIC FORM**
> • More permeable
> • Crosses skin, BBB/CNS
> $T_{1/2}$ Long because accumulates in spleen, liver, kidney, marrow, CNS, bone, and teeth
> **TOXICITY**
> 1. Displaces essential trace minerals
> 2. Covalently bonds to functional groups of proteins (-OH, -SH, -NH) → toxic
> 3. Protective peptides: Glutathione and Metalothione

CHELATORS	ADMINISTRATION	METALS	SIDE EFFECTS
DIMERCAPROL [380] **(BAL)**	IM	Pb, Hg, As, Au, Cu	Inc BP°
EDETATE (EDTA) [381] **CALCIUM DISODIUM**	IM or IV	Pb, Cd	Degenerative PCT
DEFEROXAMINE [382]	IM or IV	Fe	
PENICILLAMINE [383]	Oral	Pb, Hg, Cu	Cross sensitive with PENICILLIN

DRUG INTERACTIONS	
MECHANISM	**DRUG #1**
Δ INTENSITY	PHENOBARBITAL
	SECOBARBITAL
Δ SAFETY	DIGITOXIN DIGITOXIN DIGITOXIN
Δ PHARMACOKINETICS 1. DEC ABSORPTION	NON-LIPID SOLUBLE
	LIPID SOLUBLE DRUG (Glutethimide)
	PENICILLIN
	CAFFEINE
2. INC ABSORPTION	MAO INHIBITOR
3. Δ PLASMA PROTEIN BINDING	DICUMAROL
4. INHIBITION OF BIOTRANSFORMATION	ORAL ANTIBIOTICS
	CIMETIDINE CAFFEINE
	ORAL ANTICOAGULANTS
5. ENHANCED BIOTRANSFORMATION	PHENOBARBITAL
6. INC ELIMINATION DECREASED $T_{1/2}$	ACIDIC DRUGS (Barbiturates)
	BASIC DRUGS
SUMMATION EFFECT	PHENOTHIAZINE DIPHENHYDRAMINE
SYNERGISTIC POTENTIATION	DIAZEPAM, CODEINE,
ANTAGONISM	GUANETHIDINE GUANETHIDINE GUANETHIDINE
	EPINEPHRINE

DRUG #2	DRUG INTERACTIONS
	EFFECTS
ALCOHOL	Sleepy, drowsy
ALCOHOL	Sleepy, coma
THIAZIDE DIURETIC AMPHOTERICIN B GLUCOCORTICOIDS (CORTISOL)	Thiazide or AMP B cause hypokalemia predisposed to arrhythmia by Digitoxin Must supplement with K
ACTIVATED CHARCOAL	Charcoal adsorbs drug → Dec blood levels
MINERAL OIL	Mineral Oil – ↓ Absorption of drug
GASTRIC ACID	Acid hydrolysis of Penicillin
IRON	Caffeine reduces absorption of Fe

TYRAMINE	Cheese and wine contain Tyramine, intestinal MAO
	   – breakdown Tyramine,
	MAO inhibitor allows Inc Tyramine absorption
	   → headache, hypertensive crisis

CHLORAL HYDRATE	Chloral Hydrate displaces Dicumarol from plasma protein → ↑ bleeding

METHOTREXATE	Antibiotics kill off normal GI flora which usually
	   metabolize MTX
	MTX → ↑ bleeding, marrow suppression and
	   mucosal swelling

THEOPHYLLINE THEOPHYLLINE	Cimetidine and Caffeine inhibit transformation of Theophylline – toxicity
ALLOPURINOL	↑ Anticoagulant → bleeding
WARFARIN	Phenobarbital induces Cytochrome P_{450} ↑ Warfarin metabolism – inactive
SODIUM BICARBONATE	$NaHCO_3$ makes urine basic ∴ ↑ excret of acidic drug
AMMONIUM CHLORIDE	NH_2Cl makes urine acidic ∴ ↑ excretion of basic drug

TRICYCLIC ANTIDEPRESSANTS
BENZOTROPINE
	All 4 have anticholinergic effect, synergistic action
	   even at very low conc • Visual Δ, ↑ Intraocular P°
	   (Glaucoma), severe constipation

GLUTETHIMIDE	Greatly potentiate each other → Coma
TRICYCLIC ANTIDEPRESSANTS COCAINE AMPHETAMINES	Guanethidine is an antihypertensive. TCA, Cocaine and Amphetamines antagonize Guanethidine
LIDOCAINE	↑ Anesthetic effects of Lidocaine by delaying its absorption

DRUG INTERACTION 2	
MECHANISM	**DRUG # 1**
ANTAGONISM	EPINEPHRINE
	DIPHENHYDRAMINE CIMETIDINE
RENAL INTERACTIONS	METHENAMINE
	GLOMERULAR FILTRATION ↓ WITH AGE
	LIVER FUNCTION ↓ WITH AGE
	CORTICOSTEROIDS
	HEPARIN
METALS	ZINC ZINC
	SELENIUM
INDUCTION OF CYTOCHROME P_{450}	CIGARETTES PHENOBARBITAL DIOXIN (TCDD) INSECTICIDES
INHIBITION OF CYTOCHROME P_{450}	ISONIAZID
DRUG – DRUG INTERACTIONS	BARBITURATES (Phenobarbital)
	AMPHOTERICIN B
	AMINOGLYCOSIDES
	TETRACYCLINES
GI INTERACTIONS	TETRACYCLINES
	ORAL ANTICOAGULANTS
	DIGITALIS
	DILANTIN® PRIMAQUINE
	DIGITALIS
	ACETAMINOPHEN

DRUG INTERACTION 2	
DRUG # 2	**EFFECTS**
HISTAMINE	Reverses Histamine effects EPI – Antidote in Histamine crisis EPI – Vasoconstricts, ↓ capillary permeability HIST – Vasodilates, ↑ capillary permeability
HISTAMINE HISTAMINE	Diphenhydramine binds H_1 receptors Cimetidine binds H_2 receptors
SULFA DRUGS	Methenamine → Formaldehyde (pH < 5.5) Formaldehyde precipitates Sulfa drugs
	↑ toxicity of renal excreted drugs
	↓ Albumin, plasma protein binding sites
DIABETES	Corticosteroids ↑ blood sugar
HYPERTHYROIDISM	Heparin ↑ free fatty acid, FFA competes with Thyroxine for its receptors: ↑ Thyroxine
CADMIUM MERCURY	Zinc induces synthesis of Metalothione ↑ chelation of Cd^{++} and Hg^{++} → ↓ toxicity
	Important for synthesis of Glutathione Peroxidase
BENZOAPYRINE	All 4 ↑ the activity of Cytochrome P_{450} Benzoapyrine (BAP) → carcinogenic
DILANTIN®	INH inhibits the metabolism of Dilantin, especially in slow metabolizers
NARCOTICS (Morphine)	Inactivate each other
SALINE	Saline precipitates Amphotericin B
β-LACTAMS	Inactivate each other
ASCORBIC ACID	Fanconi's Syndrome
Di-CATION (Mg^{++}, Ca^{++}, Al^{++})	Chelate Tetracycline → ↓ absorption
AMINOGLYCOSIDES	Aminoglycoside kills GI flora → ↓ Vit K synthesis → hypoprothrombinemia, bleeding
CATHARTIC (Mg^{++}, MOM)	Hypokalemia, digitalis arrhythmia
ORAL CONTRACEPTIVE ORAL CONTRACEPTIVE	↓ Folic acid synthesis → megaloblastic anemia
ANTICHOLINERGIC	Anticholinergic → ↓ GI motility ↑ absorption and Digitalis toxicity
PROPRANOLOL	Propranolol – ↓ blood flow to liver → ↓ metabolism, ↑ toxicity. Antidote: Acetylcysteine

DRUG INTERACTIONS 3	
MECHANISM	**DRUG # 1**
ENZYME DRUG INTERACTION	COUMADIN COUMADIN (anticoagulant)
	DILANTIN®
	PHENOBARBITAL
	PHENOBARBITAL ETHANOL
	ETHANOL
	CYCLOPHOSPHAMIDE
	6-MERCAPTOPURINE
URICOSURIC	THIAZIDE DIURETIC
THERAPY	METHOTREXATE

DRUG INTERACTIONS 3	
DRUG # 2	**EFFECTS**
BARBITURATES GLUTETHIMIDE	Induces metabolism ↑ Coumadin metabolism (breakdown)
PHENOBARBITAL	Phenobarb induces enzyme / metabolism ↑ Dilantin metabolism → ↓ effect
PHENOBARBITAL	Induces Cyto P_{450} and its own metabolism
HYPERBILIRUBINEMIA	Phenobarb induces enzymes to help reduce unconjugated bilirubin (newborn)
BARBITURATES	Together induce d amino levulinic acid synthesis → ↑ porphyrin synthesis
METHANOL	Ethanol (IV) combats Methanol poisoning if given early enough. Competes for Enzs Alc dehydrogenase and Ald dehydrogenase. Ethanol has a higher affinity. Methanol → Formald → Formic acid formic acid: blindness, death Ethanol → acetald → acetic acid
CORTISOL	Cortisol inhibits Cyto P_{450} from activating Cyclo P → toxic aldophos
ALLOPURINOL	6 MP – Metab by xanthine oxidase (inactive) Allopurinol – inhibits xanthine oxidase → ↑ 6 MP → marrow suppression
↑URIC ACID Tx : PROBENECID Tx : ALLOPURINOL	Gout ↑ Uric acid secretion, blocks reabsorption, blocks xanthine oxidase, ↓ Uric acid synth
FOLATE	MTX inhibits thymidine and purine synthesis by blocking folate reductase. Folate "Rescues" cells. Folinic Acid – better, bypasses metabolism.

RADIATION

IONIZING RADIATION
- Dose dependent
- Pulls e^- from outer shells, "Ionizes"
- Radioprotective • Dec pathology of radiation
- Radiosensitive • Inc effect of radiation
- RAD: 1 Rad = 100 Ergs Energy/gm tissue
- GRAY: 1 Gy = 100 Rads = 1 J energy/kg tissue

LINEAR ENERGY TRANSFER
(LET) = KeV/μm
Inc LET → Inc destruction   Inc atomic weight → Inc LET
Uranium > carbon > α > proton > neutron > e^- > γ

GAMMA EMITTERS
- Nuclear Medicine
- Penetrate well, little/no ionization

CELLS IN MITOSIS
Highly susceptible
Rapidly dividing tissue:
- GI – electrolyte loss, leak from GI
- Marrow – infection, Dec blood cells (LØ)
- Gonads – sterility (> 4 Gy)

DOSE
1. 6 Gy • whole body irradiation
- LD50 = 8 days
- Spread dose out → tolerated better
- 1° affects bone marrow – suppression
2. 9 Gy – LD50 = 3-5 days • GI and marrow affected
3. 100 Gy – LD50 = hours • CNS: brain swells → death

FREE RADICALS H^0, OH^0, O_2^0
OH^0 is the most dangerous
Inc O_2^0 tension of tissue → Inc radicals formed and damage done

RADICALS
1. Split disulfide bonds
2. React with sulfhydryl groups
3. Fatty acid peroxidation – membrane permeability
4. DNA – very sensitive

RADIATION
1. Damage to mitosis   3. Neoplastic Δ
2. Mutation Δ   4. Cell Membrane Δ

TYPE	COMPONENT	LET	DAMAGE	PERMEABILITY
α (alpha)	He nucleus	Highest LET	More destruction	Least perm μm
β (beta)	Electron	Lower LET	Less destruction	Less perm mm
γ (gamma)	Electromagnetic	Lowest LET	Least destructive	Permeable

RADIATION

RADIOPROTECTIVE	THIOUREA	CYSTEINE CYSTEAMINE	AMINO ETHYL TRANSFERASE	ETHIOFOS	METALLOTHIONEIN
SULFHYDRYL COMPOUNDS	High dose during radiation • Dec damage • NOT effective in humans	NOT effective because dose is NOT tolerated DFR = 2	More potent protector People become ill NOT used	WR 2721 • Has phos and sulf Selective protection • NOT taken up by neoplastic cells	Natural compound • Heavy metal toxicity Radioprotective Tolerated at high doses

RADIOSENSITIVE	DACTINOMYCIN	CISPLATIN	METRONIDAZOLE (FLAGYL®)	MISONIDAZOLE
	Enhances radiation Tx: 1. Wilm's Tumor • children 2. Rhabdomyosarcoma 3. Kaposi's sarcoma	Enhances radiation	Inc sensitivity and destruction of central anoxic cells Need high doses • NOT tolerated	Metronidazole derivative SIDE EFFECT Axonal damage

SUPEROXIDE DISMUTASE

• Naturally occurring Oxy scavenger
$$O_2^0 \rightarrow O_2$$
• Inhibiting this enzyme will Inc sensitivity to radiation

PRESCRIPTION WRITING [384]

<u>DIRECTIONS</u>
1. **Name, address,** and **age** of patient
2. **Date:** Can NOT be renewed past 6 months
3. **Superscription:** Rx – Designates paper as prescription
4. **Inscription:** Name of drug and amount – dose per tablet/capsule
5. **Subscription:** Pharmacist's directions – how the drug is to be prepared and in what form
6. **Signature:** Patient's directions – quantity, frequency, mode of administration, what drug is for
7. **Renewal Instructions:** Must fill out, renew or NOT, If so – how many times
8. **Generic Substitution**
9. **DEA # and doctor's signature**

Drugs are classified into Schedules by abuse potential:

Schedule II – Written in Ink, Can NOT Refill, Must Follow Up

Schedule III or IV – Can Prescribe Orally (phone), Can Refill up to 5 times, NO more than 6 months past date

Schedule V – O.T.C. drugs, do NOT need a prescription

Drug can be both Prescribed and O.T.C.: e.g., Meclozine or Ibuprofen.

Use Brand Name, NOT Generic Name.

Use metric and decimal line (NOT Apothecary – old fashioned).

Avoid household measures – NOT precise.

Prescribe just enough to cover until next office visit.

Pharmacist must call in to alter Rx, to refill – final check.

Prescription required for Legend drugs and All Medicaid drugs (even O.T.C.).

MAC – Maximum Allowable Cost – of a drug for a Medicaid patient.

18% of prescriptions are NOT filled

25% of antiepileptics are NOT used

PRESCRIPTION WRITING [384]

CLASS	ABUSE	DEPENDENCE	EXAMPLE	PHONE	REFILL
I	HIGH	NOT ACCEPTABLE FOR MEDICAL USE	MARIJUANA HEROIN, LSD	NO	NO
II	HIGH	PSYCHOLOGICAL PHYSICAL	BARBITURATES MORPHINE	NO	NO
III	LESS THAN II	MORE PSYCHOLOGICAL	CODEINE	YES	YES
IV	LESS THAN III	LIMITED	ALPRAZOLAM	YES	YES
V	LESS THAN IV	LIMITED	TYLENOL® WITH CODEINE, O.T.C.	YES	YES

Roberta Anyone, MD
37 East Main St.
Tampa, Florida 33612
(813) 555-0000
DEA# 1234567

Name: _____   Age: _____
Address: _____   Date: _____

Rx   Ritalin Tablets   20 mg
            #80
     Sig: One tablet by mouth every 6 hrs (or $\curlyvee$ PO q 6 hrs)

     Substitution permitted____   Do Not Substitute____

     Refill ____ times   _____ MD

$\curlyvee$ = 1

$\ddot{\pi}$ = 2

$\curlyvee\ddot{\iota\iota}$ = 3

$\curlyvee\ddot{\iota\iota\iota}$ = 4

$\curlyvee\ddot{\iota\iota\iota\iota}$ = 5

IMMUNOSUPPRESSION	AZATHIOPRINE (AZT) [402]
	Metabolized to 6-MP (active) • 6-mercaptopurine Kill immunocompetent cells

MECHANISM	2 sites:
	1. Inhibits *de novo* purine synthesis – 1st step
	    Inhibits RNA & DNA synthesis
	2. Inhibits biotransformation of inosinic acid →
	    adenine & guanine
	Not specific
	Inhibits any LØ, all immune cells, all rapidly dividing
	    (mitotic) cells

METABOLISM	Well absorbed Metabolized by xanthine oxidase: 6-MP → thiouric acid ALLOPURINOL • inhibits xanthine oxidase • 2° Inc 6-MP, toxicity
USES	1. Prevents graft rejection 2. Rheumatoid arthritis 3. Renal SLE 4. Acute glomerulonephritis Administered with PREDNISONE

SIDE EFFECTS	1. 2° infection
	2. Toxicity:
	  a. marrow suppression
	  b. hepatic dysfunction
	  c. nausea, vomiting, diarrhea

Total Body Irradiation

• may die of 2° infection
• still used for bone marrow
  transplant treatment

T helper cell – Class II HLA Ag, CD_4

T cytotoxic cell – Class I HLA Ag, CD_3

CYCLOSPORINE [403]	PREDNISONE [404]
Oral $T_{1/2}$ Peak = 2 – 4 hr, 11 amino acid cyclic peptide	Dec number of LØ in spleen & lymph nodes Interferes cell cycle activated LØ Cytotoxic to T & B cells, Dec Ab NOT specific
1. Selectively inhibits IL-2 proliferation of LØ (Th & Tc) 2. Affects gene activated functional proteins 3. PMNs – NOT affected 4. Inhibits MØ indirectly by interfering with Ag interaction For normal LØ proliferation • Ca⁺⁺ is needed • CYCLOSP interferes with the protein, calmodulin in LØ DILTIAZEM • Ca⁺⁺ channel blocker potentiates CYCLOSPORINE	**ANTI-LØ GLOBULIN (ALG)**
1. Selectively inhibits IL-2 proliferation of LØ (Th & Tc) 2. Affects gene activated functional proteins 3. PMNs – NOT affected 4. Inhibits MØ indirectly by interfering with Ag interaction For normal LØ proliferation • Ca⁺⁺ is needed • CYCLOSP interferes with the protein, calmodulin in LØ DILTIAZEM • Ca⁺⁺ channel blocker potentiates CYCLOSPORINE	Interferes with early recognition NOT specific Produced from horses • may be antigenic • administ IV with PREDNISONE
Taken up by RBC, greater than 15 metabolites Metab 1° by Cyto P_{450}, demethylation, hydroxylation Excreted 1° in the bile, very little through the kidney Bioavailability Inc during Tx because it induces its own metabolism, therefore, Dec dose	**ANTI-THROMBOCYTE GLOBULIN**

1. Kidney, liver, heart transplant
    One year survival = 80 – 90%
    (Long term survival: NOT any better than AZP,
    Prednisone, ALG – all merge due to nephrotoxicity)
2. Psoriasis   4. Glomerulonephritis
3. IDDM, NIDDM   5. Rheumatoid arthritis
	Muromonab-CD3
	Murine monoclonal Ab
	Acts on T3 Ag, Use 10 – 14 days
	Severe SE: 1. Severe pulmonary
	   edema 2. Fever, chills 3. Dyspnea

1. Kidney, liver, heart transplant
    One year survival = 80 – 90%
    (Long term survival: NOT any better than AZP,
    Prednisone, ALG – all merge due to nephrotoxicity)
2. Psoriasis   4. Glomerulonephritis
3. IDDM, NIDDM   5. Rheumatoid arthritis
	METHOTREXATE

1. Kidney, liver, heart transplant
    One year survival = 80 – 90%
    (Long term survival: NOT any better than AZP,
    Prednisone, ALG – all merge due to nephrotoxicity)
2. Psoriasis   4. Glomerulonephritis
3. IDDM, NIDDM   5. Rheumatoid arthritis
	Inhibit DHF reductase
	TX: autoimmune disorders

Diarrhea, liver failure, hypertension, hirsutism,
tremors, gingival hyperplasia, nephrotoxicity
 	
PEDIATRIC LIVER TRANSPLANT
 • Need higher dose
 • Single PreOp IV dose 5 mg/kg
 • Monitor for anaphylaxis, Rx with EPI 1/1000 IV
 • Switch to oral if NO anaphylaxis
 • Most in fat, less in blood (RBC 50%, LØ 4 – 9%)
 	
TOXICITY
1. Nephrotoxic – acute tubular necrosis
2. Hepatotoxic – reversible
3. Lymphoma – seen with immunosuppression
    • regresses if Dec dose
4. Infection – 1° viral: CMV & Herpes
    (PMNs spared)
5. Convulsions
6. HT – DILTIAZEM will Inc CYCLOSPORINE
    effect without Inc nephrotoxicity
 	
NEPHROTOXICITY
 • First 4 – 6 months after any transplant
 • Usually reversible, dose related
 • Monitor CPK, BUN (usually increase)
CYCLOSPORINE → Inc TBX → Dec PGI_2
 → constricts renal arterioles → ischemia
 → defect in glomerulus and its GFR
	DRUG INTERACTIONS – CYCLOSPORINE
	1. Interfere with CYCLOSP
	    metabolism by inhibiting
	    Cyto P_{450} → Inc CYCLOSP
	    a. KETOCONAZOLE
	    b. ERYTHROMYCIN
	    c. DANAZOL
	    d. NORETHINDRONE
	    e. METHYLPREDNISOLONE
	    f. CORTISOL
	
	2. Inc metab & Inc P_{450}→ Dec CYCLOSP
	    a. PHENYTOIN
	    b. PHENOBARBITAL
	    c. RIFAMPIN
	    d. ISONIAZID (also Dec P_{450})
	    e. TRIMETHOPRIM
	    f. SULFADIMIDINE
	
	3. Change renal function
	    a. AMINOGLYCOSIDES
	    b. AMPHOTERICIN B
	    c. TRIMETHOPRIM
	      •Not nephrotoxic but does
	        interfere with excretion
	    d. TRIMETHOPRIM /
	       SULFAMETHOXAZOLE

NUTRITION (FOOD - DRUG INTERACTIONS)

MODIFICATION OF ABSORPTION
1. Δ pH, Stomach emptying time
2. Lipid solubility
3. Non-absorbable complexes
4. Δ transport processes
5. Malabsorption
6. Δ Intestinal flora

FOOD DELAYS ABSORPTION OF
AMOXICILLIN
SULFA DRUGS
ASA, ACETAMINOPHEN
DIGOXIN
FUROSEMIDE
POTASSIUM

FOOD REDUCES ABSORPTION OF
PENICILLINS
TETRACYCLINES
ASA
LEVODOPA
RIFAMPIN
DOXYCYCLINE
ISONIAZID
PHENOBARBITAL

PENICILLIN
- Acid destroys it

TETRACYCLINE
- Dairy products (Ca)
  chelates • Dec absorption

TETRACYCLINE
- Temporarily stunts growth by
  binding Ca++

LIPID SOLUBLE DRUGS
- Inc absorption with high fat diet

CHOLESTYRAMINE
- Binds bile in GI
- Interferes with Cholesterol absorption
  → Dec Vit A, D, E, K absorption
- Binds Digoxin

ORAL CONTRACEPTIVES
- Interferes with polyglutamic folate
  absorption

MONOAMINES
PHE → TYR → DOPA → DA → NE → EPI
- Found in food, but Metab by MAO in GI
- MAO inhibitors – allow these to act

LEVODOPA
- Tx Parkinsonism, crosses BBB
- "On - Off" phenomenon assoc with meals
- High protein diet induces tremors –
  large neutral amino acids compete with
  LEVODOPA for transport proteins

LAXATIVES
- NOT effective for weight loss
- Still absorb calories

DRUGS CAUSING MALABSORPTION
NEOMYCIN, KANAMYCIN
CHLORTETRACYCLINE
COLCHICINE, PHENINDIONE
PARA-AMINO SALICYLIC ACID
INDOMETHACIN, METHOTREXATE
CALCIUM SALTS
CHOLESTYRAMINE
LIQUID PARAFFIN (Mineral Oil)

MAO INHIBITORS
TRANYLCYPROMINE
PHENELZINE
PARGYLINE
- Antihypertensive medicines

Certain Foods Inc hypertension:
  aged cheese, liver, bananas, herring,
  broad beans, licorice, yeast

MAOI – Inc NE → vasoconstrict → Inc BP°

Banana peel, avocado, pineapple – high in
  amines

Fermented foods high in tyramine
  (bacterial origin) cheese, beer, wine,
  yeast, fish, liver

Broad beans – high in DA

NUTRITION (FOOD - DRUG INTERACTIONS)

<u>TRYPTOPHAN</u>
- Pyridoxal Phosphate (Vit B_6)
- Important for TRYPTOPHAN metabolism
- B_6 deficiency
- Inc side products formed

<u>ORAL CONTRACEPTIVES</u>
- Cause Dec in Vit B_6 → Dec 5-HT
  → depression
- Supplement B_6
- OC Deplete B_6 by Inc cortisol
  production

<u>ANTICONVULSANTS</u>
1. Dec folic acid
2. Coagulation defect
3. Metabolic bone disease
   - Vitamin deficiency
4. CT disorder
5. Liver enzymes induced
6. Endocrine effects

Anticonvulsants → induce Cyto P_{450} →
Inc Vit D metabolism → inactivated

Epileptic → anticonvulsant → Hypo Ca
    ↑   ↓
  Epilepsy worsens ← Osteomalacia

Cycle propagates and becomes worse

<u>PHENYTOIN</u>
- May interfere with Vit D_3 receptors

<u>PHENACETIN</u>
- Broiled beef
  · Dec PHENACETIN, destroyed
- Brussels sprouts / cabbage
  · Dec PHENACETIN absorption

<u>HIGH PROTEIN DIETS</u>
- Dec $T_{1/2}$ ANTIPYRINE and
  THEOPHYLLINE

<u>BROCCOLI</u>
Antagonizes Warfarin in 2 ways
1. Contains a lot of Vit K
2. Induces Cytochrome P_{450}
   (Also: lettuce, cabbage, spinach,
   turnip greens)

<u>RITALIN</u>•
- Dec growth in hyperactive child
- Dec appetite → dec food intake

<u>DILANTIN</u>•
- Dec folate → macrocytosis
  DO NOT supplement folate – epilepsy

<u>FOLIC ACID</u>
- Ingested – polyglutamic form
- Absorbed – monoglutamic form

O.T.C. DRUGS PAIN RELIEVERS

	ASPIRIN [392]	ACETAMINOPHEN [393]	IBUPROFEN [394]	
Cost/Dose	2¢	5.6¢	7¢	ANACIN 3® is acetaminophen
Equivalent Dose	650 mg	650 mg	200 mg	NO benefit to pain relief if take more than ceiling dose
Ceiling Dose	650 mg	650 mg	400 mg	• except with arthritis
Dysmenorrhea	++	++	+++	
Anti-Inflammatory	+++	0	+++	
Gastric Bleeding	+++	0	++	
Antipyretic	+++	+++	+++	
	CONTRAINDICATED • History • Children (Reye's)	NO ASA SIDE EFFECTS Toxic dose → hepatic destruction		

COLD REMEDIES

DRISTAN®	**NYQUIL®**
DECONGESTANT: 5 mg PHENYLEPHRINE • dose is too small to be effective ANTIHISTAMINE: CHLORPHENIRAMINE • NOT effective against viral colds • anticholinergic, does dry mucous membranes CAFFEINE – offsets sedation of antihistamine ACETAMINOPHEN • pain relief • only useful ingredient	ACETAMINOPHEN 100 mg DOXYLAMINE 75 mg PSEUDOEPHEDRINE (decongestant) DEXTROMETHORPHAN 3 mg (cough suppressant) ETHANOL 50 Proof (25%)

Ingredients

DECONGESTANTS (Sympathomimetic)

PHENYLEPHRINE [395]	PHENYLPROPANOLAMINE [396]	PSEUDOEPHEDRINE [397]
Need > 40 mg for effective dose **SIDE EFFECT** cardiac and hypertension at this dose	Low safety margin > 75 mg – hypertension Found in DEXATRIM®	Best decongestant Found in SUDAFED® Less CNS Stim than EPHEDRINE (Ephedrine – a potent CNS stimulant)

PEPTIC ULCER DISEASE

GENERAL	SODIUM BICARBONATE [398]	ANTACIDS		
		ALUMINUM SALTS [399]	CALCIUM SALTS [400]	MAGNESIUM SALTS [401]

3 FACTORS INVOLVED
Acid, Pepsin, Mucus
 	
PROMOTERS OF PEPTIC ULCERS
1. caffeine & xanthines
  → Inc cAMP → Inc acid
2. alcohol → Inc acid production
  → Dec mucus production
3. antiinflammatory drugs
  → Dec mucus production
  • ASA, Salicylates, Cortisone
  Indomethacin, Phenylbutazone
4. smoking → Stim nicotinic receptors
 	
ANTAGONISTS OF PEPTIC ULCERS
1. sedatives
2. cholinergic blockers
3. H_2 blockers – 1° therapy (CIMETIDINE)
4. antacids
 	
Vagal Stim – Inc acid and pepsin
Humeral Stim – food, protein, alcohol
Mucus – protective function
	Very effective
	• 120 ml 0.1 N HCL
	Well absorbed
	
	PROBLEM
	1. Short acting because it raises gastric pH > 7 stomach empties if pH > 4
	2. CO_2 – may cause perforation
	3. Na^+ – hypertension problems
		Poor Absorption
		1. Neutralizes more acid (250 ml)
		2. Inhibits pepsin independent of pH
		Does NOT buffer > 4
		NO emptying
		Longer acting
		
		SIDE EFFECT
		constipation
			Poor absorption
			Neutralizes acid (250 ml)
			
			SIDE EFFECT
			constipation
				SIDE EFFECT
				laxative

Ca and Mg salt antacids are used in combination to offset each other's side effects

OTHER LAXATIVES: Sodium carboxy-methyl cellulose laxative

ALCOHOL

ETHANOL [385]

KINETICS
- Water soluble
  Vd = 0.7 l/kg (= body water)
- 100% bioavailability
  90% oxidized in liver
  10% excreted in kidneys
  $0°$ kinetics (independent of conc or time)
- Elimination Rate 7 –10 g/hr

METABOLISM
1. Alcohol and acetaldehyde dehydrogenase – low amount
   a. Oxidation: alcohol DH
      ethanol → acetaldehyde (rate limiting)
   b. Acetaldehyde DH (disulfiram inhibits)
      Acetaldehyde → acetate or AcCoA
   c. Acetate → $CO_2 + H_2O$
2. Microsomal enzymes – mixed function oxidase
   a. Ethanol → polar metabolites
   b. Main pathway for high conc alcohol
   c. Drugs that induce the microsomal enzs
      → Inc the clearance of alcohol
      (e.g. PHENOBARB – Inc metab alcohol)
3. Disulfiram reaction – Antabuse®
   - Inhibits acetald DH → Inc acetaldehyde
   - Causes nausea and vomiting

EFFECTS
Local:
- Precipitate and dehydrate cytoplasm
- Mucosal irritant
- 95% Sol'n – dries up cold sores
- 70% Sol'n – bacteriocidal

SYSTEMIC
$1°$ Affects CNS
1. Inc fluidity, Dec viscosity of plasma membrane
2. Release of inhibitory control (behavior & speech)
3. Depress reticular activating system
   - Δ receptor function
   - Inc number of GABA receptors

MODERATE ALCOHOL CONSUMPTION
1. Euphoria, relieves dysphoria, Inc confidence
2. Impaired thoughts, disorganization
3. Fine discrimination, memory, insight, and concentration are diminished
4. Impaired motor coordination and visual acuity
5. Uncontrolled mood swing and emotions
6. Reduced perception of pain and fatigue

Blood Alc Conc	Effect
100 mg/dl	Dizzy / Delightful
200 mg/dl	Drunk / Disorderly
300 mg/dl	Dead Drunk
400 mg/dl	Death Risk

SIDE EFFECTS
GI tract:
1. Suppression of secretion and motility
2. Pylorospasm
3. Nausea, vomiting
4. Gastritis
5. Peptic ulcer with hemorrhaging

HEPATIC
1. Inc NADH:NAD
2. Dec gluconeogenesis → hypoglycemia
3. Ketoacidosis
4. Fatty liver
5. Alcohol hepatitis
6. Cirrhosis with ascites

CNS
1. Polyneuropathy
2. Alcohol amblyopia
3. Cerebral or cerebellar structural Δ
   - Dec motor and intellect functions
4. Wernicke's encephalopathy
5. Korsakoff's psychosis
6. Emotional problems
7. Hallucination / delirium
8. Delirium tremens

OTHER
1. Mild Anemia: folic acid deficiency
2. Alcoholic cardiomyopathy
3. Hyperemia and edema
4. Ethanol + barbiturates
   → Inc porphyrins

ALCOHOL

ETHANOL [385]

SEVERE PSYCHOLOGICAL DEPENDENCE

MEDICAL COMPLICATIONS
1. Direct effect of alcohol
2. Indirect effect of being intoxicated
3. Nutritional deficiency

TOLERANCE
Develops only in mild or moderate
    drinking
• Inherited, pharmacodynamic, and
    metabolic
• Lethal dose is same in an alcoholic as
    in nondrinkers

WITHDRAWAL
3 Stages
1. Shakes, weakness, sweating, anxiety,
    headache, nausea, intense craving
    for alcohol or sedative drugs
2. Grand mal seizures (some) by
    2nd – 3rd day → status epilepticus
3. Delirium tremens
    • auditory, visual, and tactile
      hallucinations
  Mortality rate is 10%
  Death: hyperthermia, periph vascular
    collapse or self-inflicted injury

THERAPY
1. Prevent DT with cross tolerance agents
    (PENTOBARBITAL, CHLORAL HYDRATE,
    PARALDEHYDE, CHLORDIAZEPOXIDE)
2. Vitamin injection, antibiotics,
    electrolyte balance
3. Prevent respiratory depression,
    aspiration of vomit
4. Support cardiovascular

DISULFIRAM [386]

For Patients willing to take it.

• "Acetaldehyde Syndrome:" nausea,
vomiting, flushing, hypotension,
anxiety, palpitations.

SIDE EFFECTS arrhythmia, acute heart
failure, MI, cardiovascular collapse,
respiratory depression, convulsions,
loss of consciousness

ETHANOL is used therapeutically
to treat methanol poisoning

DRUG ABUSE	METHADONE [387]	OPIOIDS / OPIATES GENERAL [388]	HEROIN [389]	MARIJUANA [390]	COCAINE [391]
ABUSED DRUGS Narcotics (opioids) CNS depressants • sedative/ hypnotic • anti-anxiety Amphetamines Cocaine Hallucinogens Marijuana	Oral, well absorbed Long duration Successful in Tx of heroin abuse Blocks heroin effects Due to availability Methadone is abused **TREATMENT GOALS** 1. Return to work 2. Stop criminal behavior 3. Social reinforcement 4. Encourage goals	<u>NATURAL</u> MORPHINE CODEINE <u>SEMISYNTHETIC</u> HEROIN HYDROMORPHONE OXYCODONE METHADONE MEPERIDINE Meperidine (Demerol®) is the only opiate to dilate pupils. <u>SYMPTOMS</u> • Dec HR • Bronchoconstriction • Constricted Pupils <u>ANTAGONIST</u> NALOXONE NALTREXONE PENTAZOCINE • Cause withdrawal symptoms	Diacetylmorphine <u>SYMPTOMS</u> 1. Potent analgesic 2. Cough suppression 3. Sedation 4. Sleepiness 5. Euphoria (IV) 6. Nausea, constipate 7. Miosis (constriction) 8. Bronchoconstriction 9. Resp depression <u>WITHDRAWAL</u> Opposite symptoms <u>COMPLICATIONS</u> 1. IV – AIDS 2. OD • acute pulm edema • cardiac failure 3. Chronic • bact endocarditis • hepatitis	2nd most widely abused drug (after alcohol) Minimal dependence <u>EFFECTS</u> 1. Mild euphoria 2. Perception Δ (time) 3. Mild symp activator • dilated pupils • Dec blood sugar • Inc appetite • conjunctiva red <u>KINETICS</u> THC • active ingredient • readily absorbed • onset 5 – 10 min Lasts 30 min Psych & cardiovasc Δ $T_{1/2}$ = 19 hr Metab $T_{1/2}$ = 50 hr Complete elimination takes 30 days	1° psychic dependence Little physical dependence Little tolerance <u>EFFECTS</u> CNS – euphoria, alertness, excitable, agitated, convulsions Sympathetic – tachycardia, arrhythmia, mydriasis, HT, vasoconstriction • Inc NE and DA release, prevents reuptake Toxic level – vent tachycardia Tx: CHLORPROMAZINE • blocks NE, DA ANTI-PSYCHOTICS MELLARIL® <u>ELIMINATION</u> renal AMMONIUM CHLORIDE Ion Trap – acid urine to Inc excretion of alkaloids: (Cocaine, Heroin, Morphine Codeine, Amphetamine)

Schedule I Drugs – NO medical use (Heroin, LSD, Marijuana, Mescaline).
Schedule II Drugs – Highly addictive, but used for Rx (Cocaine, Codeine, Morphine, Amphetamine).

DEPENDENCE
1. Psychic: compulsive drug-seeking behavior, personal satisfaction, mild habituation, severe dependence.
2. Physical: Δ physiology (neuro adaptation), withdrawal if remove drug.
3. Tolerance: Dec response to a repeated dose.
4. Cross Tolerance.

Pharmacokinetics Equations

$$Keq = \frac{CD}{AB} = \frac{Products}{Reactants}$$

$$V = \frac{Vmax\,[S]}{Km + [S]}$$

$$E = \frac{Emax\,[D]}{Kd + [D]}$$

$$y = \frac{Mx}{K + x} \qquad \frac{1}{y} = \frac{1}{m} + \frac{K}{m}\left(\frac{1}{x}\right)$$

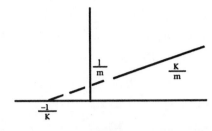

$$\% = gm/ml \qquad 2\% = \frac{2\,gm}{100\,ml} \qquad 1:1000 = \frac{1\,gm}{1000\,ml}$$

$$\frac{V}{WH} = L$$

$$[DR] = \frac{[Dt]\,[Rt]}{Keq + [Dt]}$$

$$Therapeutic\ Index = \frac{LD\,50}{ED\,50}$$

$$Safety\ Index = \frac{LD\,01}{ED\,99}$$

Effect α [DR]   (occupied R)
Emax α [Rt]

$$Effect = E = \frac{Emax\,[D]}{Kd + [D]}$$

$$\frac{1}{E} = \frac{1}{Emax} + \frac{Kd}{Emax}\left(\frac{1}{D}\right) \qquad y = a + bx$$

$$pKa = pH + \log\frac{P}{NP}$$

$$\frac{1}{E} = \frac{1}{Emax} + \left(\frac{Kd}{Emax}\right)\left(1 + \frac{I}{Ki}\right)\left(\frac{1}{D}\right)$$

Competitive Inhibition (Δ Kd)

$$\frac{1}{E} = \frac{1}{Emax}\left(1 + \frac{I}{Ki}\right) + \left(\frac{Kd}{Emax}\right)\left(1 + \frac{I}{Ki}\right)\left(\frac{1}{D}\right)$$

Noncompetitive Inhibition
(Δ Slope) (Δ Emax)

$$E = \frac{\alpha\,Emax\,[D]}{Kd + [D]} \qquad Intrinsic\ Activity = \alpha$$

$\alpha = 1$ Agonist
$\alpha < 1$ Partial Agonist

$$Vd = \frac{Q}{Co} \qquad Co = \frac{Q}{V} = \frac{Mass}{Vol}$$

Protein Binding $r = \dfrac{n[D]}{K + [D]}$

$$\frac{Dose}{mwt}\ (Avogadro's\ \#) = \#\ molecules$$

$$Css = \frac{Q}{KeVd} = \frac{Infusion}{Clearance}$$

$$f(\%) = 1 - e^{-Ket}$$

0° (saturated) $C = Co - Ke\,t$
1° $\ln C = \ln Co - K\,et$

$$Css = \frac{1}{KeVd}\binom{FD}{T} \qquad Q = D / T$$

$$f = 1 - e^{-KeTn}$$

$$t\tfrac{1}{2} = \frac{0.693}{Ke}$$

$$Clearance = KeVd = \frac{Q}{Css}$$

$$Cl = \frac{V\,[U]}{[P]} \qquad \begin{array}{l} V = Urine\ flow \\ [U] = Urine\ conc \\ [P] = Plasma\ conc \end{array}$$

REFERENCES

References from Goodman and Gilman, *The Pharmacological Basis of Therapeutics*, Ed. 8, McGraw-Hill, New York, 1990.

1. G & G pp. 192-198
2. G & G pp. 198-200
3. G & G pp. 200-201
4. G & G pp. 201-202
5. G & G p. 205
6. G & G p. 206
7. G & G p. 207
8. G & G p. 214
9. G & G p. 207
10. G & G pp. 198-200
11. G & G pp. 214, 217
12. G & G pp. 213-214
13. G & G pp. 202-203
14. G & G p. 208
15. G & G pp. 208-209
16. G & G pp. 795-796
17. G & G pp. 210-213
18. G & G p. 213
19. G & G pp. 210-213
20. G & G p. 417
21. G & G pp. 224-225
22. G & G pp. 225-226
23. G & G pp. 226-228
24. G & G pp. 228-229
25. G & G pp. 208-209
26. G & G p. 229
27. G & G pp. 233-234
28. G & G p. 235
29. G & G p. 235
30. G & G pp. 234-235
31. G & G pp. 236-238
32. G & G p. 237
33. G & G pp. 235-236
34. G & G pp. 319-320, 539-545
35. G & G pp. 405-414
36. G & G pp. 866-869
37. G & G pp. 795-796
38. G & G pp. 794-795
39. G & G pp. 150-164
40. G & G pp. 167-178, 180-181, 545-549
41. G & G pp. 122-127

42. G & G p. 126
43. G & G pp. 122-127
44. G & G pp. 127-130
45. G & G pp. 131-147
46. G & G pp. 131-147
47. G & G p. 134
48. G & G p. 142
49. G & G p. 147
50. G & G pp. 132-144
51. G & G p. 142
52. G & G pp. 135-136
53. G & G pp. 135-136
54. G & G pp. 135-136
55. G & G p. 136
56. G & G pp. 150-164
57. G & G pp. 150-164
58. G & G pp. 153-162
59. G & G pp. 180-181, 545-549
60. G & G pp. 181-184
61. G & G pp. 178-182
62. G & G pp. 182-183
63. G & G pp. 799-805
64. G & G pp. 720-727, 788
65. G & G pp. 181-184, 226-228, 793-798
66. G & G pp. 760-761, 806-807
67. G & G pp. 208-209, 308, 404, 791-793
68. G & G pp. 814-836
69. G & G pp. 828-830
70. G & G pp. 828-830
71. G & G p. 814
72. G & G pp. 840-873
73. G & G pp. 840-873
74. G & G pp. 836-837
75. G & G pp. 189, 202-203, 215-216
76. G & G pp. 205, 632
77. G & G pp. 764-774
78. G & G pp. 848-857

79. G & G pp. 848-857
80. G & G pp. 848-857
81. G & G pp. 320-329, 857-861
82. G & G pp. 439-443, 857-861
83. G & G pp. 857-861
84. G & G pp. 861-863
85. G & G pp. 865-866
86. G & G pp. 866-869
87. G & G pp. 866-869
88. G & G pp. 774-780, 805-806, 869-870
89. G & G pp. 774-780
90. G & G pp. 774-780, 805-806, 869-870
91. G & G pp. 764-774
92. G & G pp. 865-866
93. G & G pp. 774-780, 805-806, 869-870
94. G & G pp. 848-857
95. G & G pp. 1313-1322
96. G & G pp. 1313-1322
97. G & G pp. 1311-1331
98. G & G pp. 1322-1325
99. G & G pp. 714-716
100. G & G pp. 716-718
101. G & G pp. 720, 786-788
102. G & G pp. 721-725
103. G & G pp. 725-728, 788
104. G & G pp. 211, 217, 416
105. G & G p. 414
106. G & G pp. 303-305, 346-358, 424-427 454-456, 480
107. G & G pp. 369-370
108. G & G pp. 301-303
109. G & G pp. 357-358, 444-445
110. G & G p. 357

111. G & G p. 585
112. G & G pp. 303-305, 346-358, 424-427 454-456, 480
113. G & G pp. 404-414, 422-423
114. G & G pp. 414-418, 475
115. G & G pp. 406-412, 428
116. G & G pp. 210-213
117. G & G pp. 418-422
118. G & G pp. 406-411
119. G & G pp. 618, 629
120. G & G p. 1538
121. G & G p. 253
122. G & G pp. 258, 1632-1633
123. G & G p. 258
124. G & G p. 258
125. G & G pp. 439-443, 857-861
126. G & G pp. 444-445
127. G & G pp. 406, 439, 443, 447-449
128. G & G pp. 450-453, 458-459
129. G & G pp. 449-450
130. G & G pp. 453, 459-460
131. G & G pp. 466-472
132. G & G pp. 471-472, 478
133. G & G pp. 473-475, 945
134. G & G pp. 473, 475
135. G & G pp. 472-473, 1191-1192
136. G & G pp. 472, 475
137. G & G pp. 150-164
138. G & G pp. 160, 472, 477
139. G & G pp. 160, 472, 477
140. G & G pp. 518, 586, 588
141. G & G pp. 189, 210-213, 217-218, 539-544

142. G & G pp. 619-630
143. G & G pp. 160, 357, 428
144. G & G pp. 357, 428
145. G & G pp. 357, 428
146. G & G pp. 426, 428
147. G & G p. 357
148. G & G pp. 357, 428
149. G & G pp. 357, 428
150. G & G pp. 280, 303-305, 426, 428
151. G & G pp. 357, 428
152. G & G p. 357
153. G & G p. 357
154. G & G pp. 366-367, 384, 427
155. G & G pp. 428, 518, 585-588
156. G & G pp. 229, 232-234, 780, 796-798 864-865
157. G & G p. 428
158. G & G pp. 357, 444-445
159. G & G pp. 387, 396, 966-967
160. G & G pp. 387,397
161. G & G pp. 384, 387, 397, 403-404, 926
162. G & G pp. 472, 795-796
163. G & G pp. 418-423
164. G & G pp. 553-557
165. G & G pp. 259, 262-263, 575-582, 911
166. G & G pp. 518, 583-588
167. G & G pp. 585,587
168. G & G pp. 630-632
169. G & G pp. 899-902
170. G & G pp. 56-57
171. G & G p. 57
172. G & G pp. 57, 259, 925
173. G & G pp. 253, 925-928
174. G & G pp. 384, 395, 397, 403-404, 927

175. G & G pp. 518, 585-588, 966-967, 971-972
176. G & G pp. 150-164
177. G & G pp. 549-553, 926-927
178. G & G pp. 131-135, 142-147, 167-178
179. G & G pp. 167-178
180. G & G pp. 298-300
181. G & G pp. 269-270, 272
182. G & G pp. 286-292
183. G & G pp. 292-294
184. G & G pp. 294-297
185. G & G pp. 286, 297-298
186. G & G p. 1623
187. G & G pp. 301-303
188. G & G pp. 489-504
189. G & G pp. 306, 308, 508
190. G & G p. 307
191. G & G pp. 305, 368
192. G & G pp. 303-305
193. G & G pp. 301-303
194. G & G pp. 311, 320-331, 857-861
195. G & G pp. 319-322
196. G & G pp. 321-322
197. G & G p. 321
198. G & G pp. 311, 321-322
199. G & G p. 320
200. G & G p. 320
201. G & G pp. 321, 324
202. G & G p. 321
203. G & G p. 321
204. G & G pp. 489-504
205. G & G pp. 497-504
206. G & G pp. 497, 504-507
207. G & G pp. 497, 508-509
208. G & G pp. 497, 509-510
209. G & G pp. 486-487
210. G & G pp. 497, 488, 510-513

211. G & G pp. 507, 925
212. G & G pp. 280, 305-306, 488, 497, 508
213. G & G p. 497
214. G & G pp. 488, 490
215. G & G pp. 644-654
216. G & G pp. 656-659
217. G & G pp. 654-655
218. G & G p. 477
219. G & G pp. 610-611, 911
220. G & G pp. 654-655, 659-661, 663-667
221. G & G pp. 665, 674-679, 743-747
222. G & G pp. 1053-1056
223. G & G pp. 1060, 1618
224. G & G pp. 1058-1059
225. G & G pp. 1057-1060
226. G & G p. 1061
227. G & G p. 1061
228. G & G pp. 1019, 1047-1057
229. G & G pp. 1065-1085
230. G & G pp. 1069-1075
231. G & G pp. 1069, 1078-1080, 1093
232. G & G pp. 1069 , 1075-1078
233. G & G pp. 1080-1081
234. G & G p. 1092
235. G & G p. 1093
236. G & G pp. 1085-1092
237. G & G pp. 1130-1134, 1584
238. G & G pp. 1138-1140
239. G & G pp. 1134-1136
240. G & G pp. 1140-1141
241. G & G pp. 1019, 1125-1130
242. G & G pp. 1117-1125
243. G & G pp. 1098-1113, 1153-1154
244. G & G pp. 1146-1149, 1157-1159
245. G & G pp. 1149-1152, 1157-1160
246. G & G pp. 1154, 1157

247. G & G pp. 1152-1153, 1157-1158
248. G & G pp. 1108, 1153-1158
249. G & G pp. 1019, 1111-1112, 1154-1157
250. G & G pp. 1107, 1165-1168, 1175, 1179
251. G & G pp. 1168-1169, 1174-1175
252. G & G pp. 1169-1171, 1174-1175
253. G & G pp. 1173-1174
254. G & G pp. 1178-1179
255. G & G pp. 1184-1186, 1194-1196
256. G & G pp. 1019, 1186-1187, 1195
257. G & G pp. 1187-1188, 1234
258. G & G pp. 472-473, 1191-1192
259. G & G pp. 1182-1184
260. G & G p. 1188
261. G & G pp. 988-991
262. G & G pp. 991-994
263. G & G pp. 985-987, 1052
264. G & G pp. 981-983, 1000, 1583
265. G & G pp. 987-988
266. G & G pp. 1000-1001
267. G & G pp. 1001-1002, 1585
268. G & G pp. 1117-1125
269. G & G pp. 1001-1002, 1585
270. G & G pp. 1008-1014
271. G & G p. 1003
272. G & G p. 1001
273. G & G pp. 1206, 1238-1239
274. G & G pp. 1206, 1238, 1586
275. G & G pp. 1447, 1450
276. G & G pp. 1384-1395
277. G & G pp. 1206, 1254, 1458-1459

278. G & G pp. 1207, 1256-1257, 1395-1397
279. G & G pp. 1206, 1240-1241
280. G & G pp. 1241-1244
281. G & G pp. 1244-1246
282. G & G pp. 1215-1216
283. G & G pp. 1216-1218, 1272
284. G & G pp. 1249-1251
285. G & G pp. 1223-1227, 1271-1272
286. G & G pp. 1235-1236, 1271
287. G & G pp. 1205, 1236
288. G & G pp. 1205, 1228-1230
289. G & G pp. 1205, 1230-1232
290. G & G pp. 1220-1222
291. G & G pp. 1252-1253
292. G & G p. 1248
293. G & G pp. 1239-1240
294. G & G pp. 486,   1351-1352, 1431-1436
295. G & G pp. 1343-1346
296. G & G pp. 1334-1343
297. G & G pp. 1346-1351
298. G & G p. 1350
299. G & G pp. 935-937
300. G & G p. 739
301. G & G pp. 732-733, 738-740
302. G & G pp. 473-475, 945, 1346
303. G & G pp. 881-886
304. G & G pp. 1347-1351
305. G & G pp. 1207, 1353-1354, 1395
306. G & G pp. 1353-1354
307. G & G pp. 1431-1459
308. G & G pp. 1206, 1253-1254, 1458
309. G & G pp. 1447-1450
310. G & G pp. 725-726, 1431, 1439-1441
311. G & G pp. 1447-1449, 1660

165

312. G & G pp. 1447, 1450
313. G & G pp. 1447, 1449
314. G & G pp. 725-727, 788
315. G & G pp. 1206,1253
316. G & G pp. 1206, 1254, 1458-1459
317. G & G p. 1205
318. G & G pp. 1413-1430
319. G & G p. 1422
320. G & G pp. 1413-1427
321. G & G p. 1422
322. G & G p. 1421
323. G & G pp. 1422-1423
324. G & G p. 1422
325. G & G pp. 1207, 1255-1256, 1384-1395 1402-1409
326. G & G pp. 1207, 1391-1392
327. G & G p. 1391
328. G & G p. 1391
329. G & G p. 1384
330. G & G pp. 1392, 1403-1404
331. G & G pp. 1391-1392
332. G & G pp. 1397-1409
333. G & G pp. 1402-1409
334. G & G pp. 1207, 1256-1257, 1395-1397
335. G & G pp. 1395-1397
336. G & G p. 1401
337. G & G pp. 935-937
338. G & G pp. 943, 946
339. G & G pp. 937-939
340. G & G pp. 937-939
341. G & G p. 919
342. G & G pp. 189, 206, 949-950
343. G & G pp. 205, 216, 632-634, 950
344. G & G pp. 345, 370-378, 538-539
345. G & G pp. 1463-1484
346. G & G p. 1486
347. G & G p. 1486
348. G & G p. 1486
349. G & G pp. 1484-1487

350. G & G p. 1486
351. G & G pp. 1368-1371
352. G & G p. 1371
353. G & G p. 1371
354. G & G p. 1371
355. G & G p. 1377
356. G & G pp. 1373-1377
357. G & G pp. 1367, 1379-1380
358. G & G pp. 1377-1379
359. G & G pp. 1376-1677
360. G & G p. 1364
361. G & G pp. 1503-1507
362. G & G pp. 1500, 1506-1507
363. G & G pp. 1367-1373
364. G & G pp. 1510-1517
365. G & G pp. 1501, 1507-1509
366. G & G p. 1516
367. G & G pp. 1615-1621
368. G & G p. 322
369. G & G pp. 764-774
370. G & G pp. 1622- 1623
371. G & G pp. 1622-1623
372. G & G pp. 1663-1634
373. G & G pp. 135-136, 1630
374. G & G p. 1621
375. G & G pp. 1621-1631
376. G & G pp. 1593-1598
377. G & G pp. 1598-1602
378. G & G pp. 1630-1631
379. G & G pp. 1605-1606
380. G & G pp. 1609-1611
381. G & G pp. 1607-1608
382. G & G pp. 1611-1612
383. G & G pp. 1610-1611
384. G & G pp. 1640-1647
385. G & G pp. 345, 370-379, 538-539
386. G & G pp. 378-379
387. G & G pp. 508-509, 533-534, 560-561
388. G & G pp. 485-514
389. G & G p. 500
390. G & G pp. 549-553

391. G & G pp. 319-320, 539-545
392. G & G pp. 644-653
393. G & G pp. 1267-1270, 1539, 1586
394. G & G pp. 665-668
395. G & G p. 207
396. G & G pp. 214, 217
397. G & G p. 214
398. G & G pp. 907-908
399. G & G p. 907
400. G & G p. 908
401. G & G p. 907
402. G & G pp. 1235-1236, 1270-1271
403. G & G pp. 1267-1270, 1586
404. G & G pp. 1447, 1450

ABBREVIATIONS

1°   primary
2°   secondary
5–FU   5–fluorouracil
5–HT   5–hydroxytryptamine
6–TG   6–thioguanine
α   alpha
β   beta
Δ   altered, changed

A

Ab   antibody
ABVD   adriamycin, bleomycin, vinblastine, dacarbazine
accum   accumulate
ACE   angiotensin converting enzyme
Ach   acetylcholine
AChE   acetylcholinesterase
ACTH   adrenocorticotropic hormone
ADH   antidiuretic hormone
Admin   administration
Ag   antigen
AHH   aryl hydrocarbon hydroxylase
ALL   acute lymphoblastic leukemia
AML   acute monocytic leukemia
AMOXICIL   amoxicillin
AMP B   amphotericin B
AMPH   amphetamine
ANS   autonomic nervous system
Ant Pit   anterior pituitary
Antichol   anticholinergic
anticoag   anticoagulant
Antihist   antihistamine
AP   action potential
APD   action potential depolarization, AP duration
ARA-C   Cytarabine
arrhyth   arrhythmia

Art   arterial
ASA   acetyl salicylic acid (Aspirin)
assoc   associated
AT   antithrombin
ATR   atropine
AVN   atrial ventricular (AV) node

B

b/c   because
BAL   British anti–Lewisite
BARB   barbiturate
BBB   blood–brain barrier
BDZ   benzodiazepine
BENZ   benzathine
bioavail   bioavailability
BP°   blood pressure
Br   bromine, bromide
BROMO   bromocriptine
BUN   blood urea nitrogen
BV   blood volume
BØ   basophil

C

C.A.S.T.   Cardiac Antiarrhythmic Study Trials
CA   cancer
cAMP   cyclic AMP
CBL   cerebral (cortex)
CBLLR   cerebellar
Ccr   creatinine clearance
CEPH   cephalosporins
CHF   congestive heart failure
CHLOROQ   chloroquine
CL   corpus luteum
clav   clavulanate
CLIND   clindamycin

Cmpd compound
CNS central nervous system
CO cardiac output
COMT catecholamine–o–methyl transferase
conc concentration
contract contraction
CPK creatine phosphokinase
CPZ chlorpromazine
CRF corticotropin–releasing factor
CSF cerebrospinal fluid
CT connective tissue
CTZ chemoreceptor trigger zone
CUR curare
CV cardiovascular
CYCLOSP cyclosporine
Cyt P$_{450}$ cytochrome P$_{450}$

D

D.O.C. drug of choice
DA dopamine
DAD delayed after depolarization
DCT distal collecting tubules
DDx differential diagnosis
Dec decrease
decomp decomposition
Dent dentistry
depend dependence
depol depolarization
Depr depression
DES diethylstilbestrol
DHF dihydrofolic
DHP dihydropteric
DHT dihydrotestosterone
DI diabetes insipidus
DIG digitalis
Dis disease
DISM disorder initiating and maintaining sleep (insomnia)
DIT diiodotyrosine
DM diabetes mellitus

DT delirium tremens
dv/dt change in velocity / change in time
Dx diagnosis

E

EAD early after depolarization
ECF extracellular fluid
ECT electroconvulsive therapy
EDTA edetate calcium disodium
EDV end diastolic volume
ENC encephalon
Endo endometriosis
ENT ear, nose, throat
Enz enzyme
EPI epinephrine
ERP excitation reaction potential
esp especially
EST estrogen
ETH ACID ethacrynic acid
EØ eosinophil

F

FA fatty acid
F–dUMP 5–fluoro–2'–deoxyuridine–5' phosphate
FLU flucytosine
FORMALD formaldehyde
FSH follicle–stimulating hormone

G

Gang ganglia
GB gall bladder
GC glucocorticoids
gen generation
GFR glomerular filtration rate
GH growth hormone
GI gastrointestinal
Gm gram

Gn RH gonadorelin (gonadotropin releasing hormone)
GRH growth hormone releasing hormone

H

HAL halothane
HCG human chorionic gonadotropin
HDL high–density lipoproteins
HGH human growth hormone
HGPRT hypoxanthine-guanine phophoribosyltransferase
HLA-DR2 human leukocytes antigen – DR2
HMG human menopausal gonadotropin
HR heart rate
hr hour
HT hypertension
HV herpes virus
Hyp hypnotic
hypot hypotension

I

I iodine
I* radioactive iodine
IDDM insulin dependent diabetes mellitus
IL interleukin
IM intramuscular
Inc increase
Induct induction
INH isonicotinic acid hydrazide
ISO isoproterenol
IT intrathecal
IV intravenous

K

KETO ketoconazole

L

L-ASPase L-asparaginase
LA local anesthetic
LDL low–density lipoproteins
LET linear energy transfer
LH luteinizing hormone
LHRH luteinizing hormone releasing hormone
LIDO lidocaine
LVEDV left ventricular end diastolic volume
LVESV left ventricular end systolic volume
LØ lymphocyte

M

MAC minimum alveolar concentration
MAO monoamine oxidase
MAO I MAO inhibitors
MAP mean arterial pressure
MC mineralocorticoids
Med medicine
memb membrane
metab metabolism
METH methicillin
MI myocardial infarction
min minute
MIT monoiodotyrosine
MOM milk of magnesia
MOPP mechlorethamine, oncovin, prednisone, procarbazine regimen
MRSA methicillin–resistant staphylococci
MTX methotrexate
MUSC muscarine
MØ macrophage

N

N nerve
NE norepinephrine
NEO neostigmine
NIC nicotine
NIDDM non-insulin dependent
diabetes mellitus
NIF nifedipine
NP nonprotonated
NS nervous system
NSAID nonsteroidal
antiinflammatory drugs

O

O.T.C. over the counter
OC oral contraceptives
OD overdose
Ortho orthostatic

P

P° pressure
P protonated
PAC premature atrial contraction
Parasymp parasympathetic
PAS para-aminosalicylate
PAT paroxysmal atrial tachycardia
PBP penicillin binding protein
PCT proximal collecting tubules
Peds pediatrics
PEN penicillin
PEN G penicillin G
PEN V penicillin V
Penase penicillinase
Perox peroxidase
PG prostaglandin
PGE prostaglandin E
PGI prostacyclin
PHENOBARB phenobarbital
Pheo pheochromocytoma

PIF prolactin inhibiting factor
PIH prolactin inhibiting hormone
Pit pituitary
PLT platelet
PMN polymorphonuclear neutrophil
Pneu pneumonia
PNS parasympathetic nervous system
PO per oral
POSTSYN postsynaptic
ppt precipitates
PR peripheral resistance
PRESYN presynaptic
PRH prolactin releasing hormone
PROC procaine
prod product
PROG progesterone
PROPOX propoxyphene
prot protein
Prt Bd protein bound
PSVT paradoxical supraventricular
tachycardia
Pt patient
PTH parathyroid hormone
PTU propylthiouracil
Pulm pulmonary

Q

QT QT interval on ECG
QUIN quinidine

R

RBC red blood cell
rcptr receptor
Rd radical
REM rapid eye movement
RES reserpine
RIF rifampin
Rxn reaction

S

SAL salbutamol (albuterol)
SE side effect
sed sedative
signif significant
SLE systemic lupus erythematosus
Sm smooth
SMZ sulfamethoxazole
sol soluble
Sol'n solution
SQ subcutaneous
Staph staphylococci
stim stimulate
stk stroke
Subl sublingual
SULF sulfonamide
Symp sympathetic
Synd syndrome

T

T.E.N.S. transdermal electrical neural stimulation
T4 thyroxine
Tachy tachycardia
TAG triacylglycerides, triglycerides
TB tuberculosis
Tc T cytotoxic cell
TCA tricyclic antidepressants
TEST testosterone
Th T helper cell
THC tetrahydrocannabinol
THF tetrahydrofolate
TIC ticarcillin
TIT triiodothyronine
TPA tissue plasminogen activator
TSH thyroid stimulating hormone, thyrotropin
Tx treatment
TXA thromboxane
T° temperature

U

UMP uridine monophosphate pyrophosphorylase
UT urinary tract
UTI urinary tract infection
UV ultraviolet

V

V or **Vent** ventricle
VANCO vancomycin
VBL vinblastine
VC vasoconstriction
Vd volume of distribution
vel velocity
VER verapamil
Vit vitamin
vol volume
VX vincristine

W

w/ with
w/o without
WBC white blood cell

X

x times

Y

yrs years

INDEX